HORMONE BALANCE

Natural Remedies for Women to Balance Hormones, Lose Weight, and Boost Energy

Miss Harmony

Copyright 2022 by Miss Harmony- All rights reserved.

This document is geared towards providing exact and reliable information in regard to the topic and issue covered. The publication is sold with the idea that the publisher is not required to render accounting, officially permitted, or otherwise, qualified services. If advice is necessary, legal or professional, a practiced individual in the profession should be ordered.

- From a Declaration of Principles which was accepted and approved equally by a Committee of the American Bar Association and a Committee of Publishers and Associations.

In no way is it legal to reproduce, duplicate, or transmit any part of this document in either electronic means or in printed format. Recording of this publication is strictly prohibited and any storage of this document is not allowed unless with written permission from the publisher. All rights reserved.

The information provided herein is stated to be truthful and consistent, in that any liability, in terms of inattention or otherwise, by any usage or abuse of any policies, processes, or directions contained within is the solitary and utter responsibility of the recipient reader. Under no circumstances will any legal responsibility or blame be held against the publisher for any reparation, damages, or monetary loss due to the information herein, either directly or indirectly.

Respective authors own all copyrights not held by the publisher.

The information herein is offered for informational purposes solely, and is universal as so. The presentation of the information is without contract or any type of guarantee assurance.

The trademarks that are used are without any consent, and the publication of the trademark is without permission or backing by the trademark owner. All trademarks and brands within this book are for clarifying purposes only and are the owned by the owners themselves, not affiliated with this document.

CONTENTS

1. **Introduction 7**
   - What are hormones? 7
   - Major hormones of your body and their functions 12
   - Which body tissues make hormones? 14
   - Role of hormones in female sexual and reproductive health .. 18
   - How do hormones change with age and time? 20

2. **Understanding hormone imbalance 23**
   - Why do hormones lose balance? 24
   - Signs and symptoms of hormone imbalance 30
   - Impact of hormone imbalance on female reproductive health 33
   - Most common hormonal imbalances faced by women 35

3. **Managing Hormone Imbalance 38**
   - Diet tips 39
   - Lifestyle tips 45

4. **Natural herbs and ingredients 52**
   - Minerals and nutrients 70

5. **Foods to Avoid 76**

6. **Cycle Syncing 84**
   - Why is cycle syncing important? 84
   - Who can benefit from cycle syncing? 85
   - Framework for cycle syncing 87
   - How to start cycle syncing? 88

Seed cycling for hormone imbalance 89
Cycle syncing and the Infradian rhythm 93

7. Cycle syncing for Menstrual phase 96
Hormonal changes during menstrual phase 96
Some facts you might not know about your monthly period .. 99
Optimal foods for menstrual phase 101
Phase-specific recipes... 103
Phase-specific exercises 111

8. Cycle Syncing for Follicular Phase................ 113
Hormonal changes... 113
Optimal foods for follicular phase 116
Phase-specific recipes... 118
Phase-specific exercises 127

9. Cycle Syncing for Ovulatory phase 129
Optimal foods for ovulatory phase 132
Phase-specific recipes... 134
Phase-specific exercises 145

10. Cycle Syncing for Luteal Phase 146
Hormonal changes during luteal phase.................................. 146
Optimal foods for luteal phase 148
Phase-specific recipes... 150
Phase-specific exercises 159

Conclusion 161

DISCLAIMER

The information provided in this book is the author's opinions about hormone imbalance and its management. The contents of this book are intended for educational purposes only. The author is not your medical advisor or healthcare provider. The details of this book are in no case any kind of medical advice, medical prescription or professional diet plan for managing hormone imbalance. The statements made about hormones in this book are not intended to identify, diagnose, cure, or prevent hormone imbalance or any other medical condition related to it. Please consult your medical practitioner or healthcare advisor regarding the recommendations and suggestions given in this book for managing hormone imbalance.

Understand that this book is in no case a scientific publication, medical consultation or advice and it is not meant to be a substitute for professional healthcare advice. If you or any other person experience symptoms for hormone imbalance or other medical conditions, please consult a licensed professional medical advisor such as your physician. Do not self-medicate. You must consult your physician before making any lifestyle changes or observing any diet plans to ensure that you are in a sound medical condition to follow the suggestions in this book and that the recommendations given in this book are appropriate for your personal health.

Do not disregard or ignore any professional medical advice in comparison to information given in this book. In case you feel a medical emergency or serious health concern, immediately call and consult your physician and seek urgent medical attention. The author and the publisher are not liable or responsible for any medical, physical, mental loss or negative effects arising from the use of information or recommendations provided in this book. The opinions, suggestions and recommendations given in this book are not related to those given by any medical, educational or wellness institution or online platform.

YOUR EXCLUSIVE GIFT

To thank you for your purchase, we're offering for free an exclusively gift for the readers of *Hormone Balance*.

By downloading this exclusive PDF, you will get 4 summary pages with all the recommended tips and food for each menstrual cycle phase!

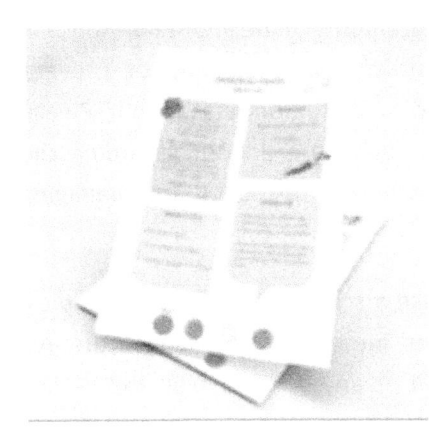

To access your gift:

- Go to the link decimobooks.com/extra-hormone

- Or scan the QR code below.

Please, don't forget to leave a review on Amazon if you like Miss Harmony! Thank you!

1. INTRODUCTION

If you are a woman and dealing with the very common female problems of hormonal imbalance and weight issues then you have picked up the right book. Here you will find all the answers to your questions of what are hormones, how they affect your body, what happens if they are imbalanced and how you can restore their balance naturally. So, if you want to be healthier and get rid of these problems then read on!

WHAT ARE HORMONES?

Hormones, also known as the chemical messengers, are molecules responsible for regulating numerous physiological functions of your body. They are released by several glands, tissues and organs in your body and this collectively makes up the endocrine system. The main function of hormones is to carry chemical signals and transport information from one organ to another via the route of blood circulation. They are extremely essential biological components without which the idea of living a healthy life seems impossible.

More than 50 hormones in the human body have been identified by science to date. Each hormone is responsible for performing a specific biological function and they control a variety of biological processes including:

- Metabolism
- Reproduction (fertility, menstrual cycle)
- Emotional health (moods)
- Homeostasis (your body's internal balance of sugar, water, blood pressure and other fluid levels)
- Growth and development
- Sexual health
- Sleep cycle

The balance of hormones in the body is what keeps you healthy and all your functions going properly. This why it is said that with hormones, a little goes a long way. Even an apparently insignificant or slight imbalance in the levels of a hormone can cause unwanted health issues and serious complications which are discussed in later chapters of this book.

HORMONES AND CELL SIGNALING

In your body, hormones perform the very important task of transporting signals from one cell to another. The kind of cell signaling performed by hormones is classified into four types depending upon how they are released and what is there target cell:

1. **Autocrine signaling:** This is when hormone acts and transports signals to the same cell that secretes it.

2. **Paracrine signaling:** This is when hormone acts on a cell very close to its secreting without the need to travel via blood circulation.
3. **Intracrine signaling:** This is when a hormone is produced within and cell it also acts within the same cell without crossing the cell boundary.
4. **Endocrine signaling:** This is when a hormone is released from a specific gland and it travels via bloodstream to transport signals to its target cell.

TYPES OF HORMONES

There is a wide variety of hormones in the human body, each having its own function and properties. However, all the hormones can be divided into three main types on the basis of their chemical composition and structure.

1. Peptide (Water-soluble) hormones

These are the hormones which are made up of long chains of amino acids which are called poly-peptide chains, hence the name peptide hormones. These hormones are hydrophilic which means they are easily soluble in water. This property renders them inability to cross cell membranes which are made up of phospholipids (water-hating molecules). However, they freely move in the blood stream and travel from one cell to another. This type includes many important hormones of the body such as insulin that is released from the pancreas, oxytocin that is released from the brain, and growth hormone and follicle stimulating hormone (FSH) that are released from the pituitary gland.

2. Steroid (Lipid-soluble) hormones

These are the hormones which are derived from cholesterol and thus are termed as steroid hormones as they contain the main structural component of steroids. There chemical structure is similar to that of cholesterol and they are soluble in lipids or fats due to which they can easily cross cell membranes. However, this property makes them unable to freely transport in the blood which is why they travel across the bloodstream with the help of transport proteins. This type includes many important reproductive hormones such as estrogen, progesterone and testosterone which are released by the reproductive organs of your body. Another very important steroid hormone is cortisol which is released by the adrenal glands in your body.

3. Amino acid-derived hormones

These hormones may seem similar to peptide hormones as they are also derived from amino acids, but actually they are different. This is because these hormones are not made up of long peptide chains rather small amino acids like tyrosine and tryptophan. An example of amino acid-derived hormones is melatonin which is the sleep-regulating hormone produced by the pineal gland in your brain. Others include the hormones epinephrine and norepinephrine which are produced by adrenal glands and thyroxine which is produced by thyroid gland.

WHAT DO HORMONES DO?

You might have already gotten the idea that hormones carry out very important bodily functions. But it is important to understand their general role in the body in detail so that you can know what is happening in your body and how it affects your health. Sometimes a hormone works alone to carry out a specific function and sometimes a chain reaction of hormones is required to accomplish a physiological task. Now, let us explain to you how hormones carry out their functions.

First you need to understand the lock and key system of hormone functioning. Just like how a key works only if it fits a lock, similarly a hormone works only if it fits a cell. Think of a hormone as a key and the target cell as a lock. If the lock has specific receptors on the cell wall that coincide with the hormone only then can the hormone function and deliver its signals to target cells leading to a specific action.

Hormones are responsible for carrying out two types of communication in your body:

1. From an endocrine gland to an endocrine gland

In this type of communication, a hormone is initially released by an endocrine gland which is used to stimulate another endocrine gland to change the balance or levels of its hormones. An example of this type of communication is when the pituitary gland releases the thyroid-stimulating hormone (TSH) which acts on the thyroid gland prompting it to release its hormones to carry out specific functions in the body.

2. From an endocrine gland to a target organ

In this type of communication, a hormone is released from an endocrine gland which then acts on a specific target organ. An example of this type of communication is the release of insulin from pancreas which acts on different muscular and liver cells to regular blood levels of glucose.

MAJOR HORMONES OF YOUR BODY AND THEIR FUNCTIONS

For knowing the balance of hormones in your body and how a disturbed hormone balance can affect your health, it is very important to know the major hormones, where they are produced and what is their function.

Hormone	Produced by	Function
Adrenocorticotropic hormone (ACH)	Pituitary gland	Regulation of sex hormones i.e., estrogen, progesterone and testosterone, production of eggs in women and sperm in men
Aldosterone	Adrenal glands	Regulation of homeostasis (balance of fluids, water, salt and blood pressure)
Corticosteroid	Adrenal glands	Maintenance of electrolyte balance, muscle strength and anti-inflammatory actions
Corticotropin releasing hormone (CRH)	Hypothalamus	Regulation of release of ACH by pituitary gland
Epinephrine	Adrenal glands	Rise in heart rate, blood flow and intake of oxygen
Erythropoietin	Kidneys	Production of red blood cells

Estrogen	Ovaries	Development of female sexual characteristics, regulation of reproductive functions, maintenance of uterine and breast functioning, effect on bone health
Follicle-stimulating hormone (FSH)	Pituitary gland	Regulation of sex hormones i.e., estrogen, progesterone and testosterone, production of eggs in women and sperm in men
Glucagon	Pancreas	Increase in blood glucose levels
Gonadotropin releasing hormone (GnRH)	Hypothalamus	Regulation of releases of LH and FSH by pituitary gland
Growth hormone (GH)	Pituitary gland	Regulation of growth and development, production of proteins, distribution of fats
Growth hormone releasing hormone (GHRH)	Hypothalamus	Regulation of release of GH by pituitary gland
Humoral factors	Thymus	Development and maintenance of lymphoid system
Insulin	Pancreas	Decrease in blood glucose levels, stimulation of muscle and liver cells to process glucose
Luteinizing hormone (LH)	Pituitary gland	Regulation of sex hormones i.e., estrogen, progesterone and testosterone, production of eggs in women and sperm in men
Melatonin	Pineal gland	Maintenance of sleep and wake cycle

Norepinephrine	Adrenal glands	Maintenance of blood pressure
Oxytocin	Pituitary gland	Contraction of uterus during pregnancy, production of milk in breasts
Parathyroid hormone	Parathyroid glands	Regulation of serum levels of calcium
Progesterone	Ovaries	Stimulation of uterine lining for egg to be fertilized, stimulation of milk ducts to produce milk
Prolactin	Pituitary gland	Initiation and maintenance of breast milk production, regulation of levels of sex hormones
Renin and angiotensin	Kidneys	Regulation of blood pressure
Thyroid-stimulating hormone (TSH)	Pituitary gland	Production and secretion of thyroid hormones
Thyrotropin releasing hormone (TRH)	Hypothalamus	Regulation of release of TSH by pituitary gland
Vasopressin (Anti-diuretic hormone)	Pituitary gland	Control of blood pressure by regulating water retention in kidneys

WHICH BODY TISSUES MAKE HORMONES?

Hormones are released by various glands or organs in your body. A gland is an organ which is responsible for releasing wither of the several body secretions i.e., hormone, tears, sweat, saliva or digestive juices. There are specialized glands in your body each responsible for secreting specific hormones. These hormone-releasing glands make up the endocrine system of your body. Let's have a look at all the glands of your endocrine system that release hormones in your body:

1. **Hypothalamus**

This is a very important gland that is present in a small region of the brain, it is connected to the pituitary gland via a pituitary stalk. It is often referred to as the smart coordinating center of your brain. It links your entire endocrine system to your nervous system. The main purpose of hypothalamus is to maintain homeostasis in your body. Homeostasis is a balance of blood pressure, blood sugar levels, salt, water and electrolytes in your body.

2. **Pituitary gland**

This gland, as small as the size of a pea, is responsible for functions as large as regulation of very vital functions of your body. It lies just below the base of your brain under the hypothalamus. The pituitary gland is divided into two lobes i.e., the anterior pituitary and the posterior pituitary. Each lobe produces different and specific hormones which carry out very important and specified functions in your body including regulation of reproductive functions, growth and development, regulation of menstrual cycle and maintenance of water balance in the body.

3. **Thyroid gland**

This butterfly-shaped gland is located just under the skin at the front of your neck. T is a very important gland in your body which is responsible for regulation the rate and speed of metabolism. This means it all depends on thyroid gland how your body processes food and consumes dietary components to produce energy. It determines how fast your body can burn calories upon physical activity and thus regulates your weight.

4. **Parathyroid gland**

As the name suggests, these glands are located behind your thyroid gland. In rare cases, they may be located in your chest around the esophagus (ectopic parathyroid glands). They are usually four in number and just the size of a pea. The parathyroid gland is responsible for releasing the parathyroid hormone which maintains the optimal level of calcium in your body.

5. **Pineal gland**

This gland is actually the smallest organ in your body. It is even smaller than the size of a pea and is located in your brain, just behind the corpus callosum which the line that connects the two hemispheres of your brain. Also called conarium, the pineal gland is responsible for releasing melatonin. This hormone regulates your sleep cycle and helps maintain a good sleeping routine.

6. **Adrenal glands**

Also known as the suprarenal glands, the adrenal glands are two triangular-shaped glands that are located one the top of your kidneys. The hormones produced by adrenal glands help regulate very important bodily functions. These include regulation of metabolism and immune functioning, maintenance of blood pressure, regulation of stress response and maintenance of heart rate.

7.   Pancreas

The pancreas is a leaf-shaped organ located just behind the stomach in your abdomen. This organ is part of both the endocrine system and the digestive system, it releases digestive enzymes that aid in digestion of food. It releases very important hormones I.e., insulin and glucagon which are responsible for maintain the levels of glucose in your body.

8.   Ovaries

Ovaries are organs that are specific to the female gender. There are two oval-shaped ovaries in a female body which are located on the two sides of her uterus just below the point where fallopian tubes open. They are one of the most important reproductive organs of a female body. The ovaries are responsible for releasing eggs for reproduction. They also release the female sec hormones estrogen and progesterone which regulate the menstrual cycle and perform other important roles like regulation of reproductive functions, development of sexual characteristics, female body shape and growth of hair

Besides all these glands, other organs in the body such as kidneys, gut, liver and fat tissue also release some hormones which carry out specific functions in the body.

ROLE OF HORMONES IN FEMALE SEXUAL AND REPRODUCTIVE HEALTH

The entire system of sex and reproduction in females is controlled and regulated by hormones. The most important reproductive hormones in the female body are estrogen, progesterone and androgens. They influence every sexual or reproductive change that occurs in your body from the start of puberty, to menopause and till death. Whether it be development of breasts, growth of body hair, getting your first period, absence of a period, having sex, getting pregnant, giving birth, menopause or any other reproductive complication in your body, each and every thing is related to and influenced by these hormones in one way or the other.

The levels of these reproductive hormones keep fluctuating during your lifetime and it impacts your sexual and reproductive health in a positive or negative way accordingly. There is a very precise shift in the levels of these hormone during different phases of your menstrual cycle, each playing its own specific role to keep your reproductive system strong and healthy. These hormones are very strongly influenced by a change in their levels caused by introducing extrinsic hormones by using birth control pills. The most dramatic shift of hormones that can occur in a female body is during pregnancy where the body temporarily develops a new organ called the placenta and releases the reproductive hormone progesterone.

The female menstrual cycle is the first thing that comes to your mind when your think of female hormones and reproduction. When we talk about the menstrual cycle you might only think of your period. But it actually goes way beyond just your period. It is entirely regulated by hormones and without these hormones your reproductive system would be like a stagnant machine with no fuel to drive it.

After understanding the role of hormones in female reproductive and sexual health, let's have a look at the specific sec hormones and their precise roles in your body:

1. **Androgens**

Usually thought to be as male-specific hormones, androgens are also produced in small amounts in females as well. They are produced by ovaries and adrenal glands and perform very important reproductive functions. Testosterone is the most important androgen produced in the female body. The absence of this hormone or imbalance in its levels can cause problems like acne, hirsutism, fatigue, loss of libido, weight gain, mood swings, irregular menstruation and even infertility.

2. **Progesterone**

Progesterone is the most important hormone when it comes to regulation of reproductive functions and pregnancy in your body. It is released by your ovaries mostly during the second half of your menstrual cycle and helps maintain menstrual balance and prepares your body for pregnancy. In the second half of the menstrual cycle, when the egg is released from ovaries, progesterone stimulates the uterine lining to become thick and prepare for implantation of the fertilized egg. This hormone is also very important during the first trimester of pregnancy as it is released b the placenta to protect the fetus and fulfill its nutritional requirements. Progesterone also stimulates development of mammary glands in breasts for milk production.

Besides its main function i.e., regulation of the menstrual cycle, estrogen also performs other bodily functions like maintenance of bone health by bone development and regulation of several cardiac, urinary and vascular functions in females. You may be even more interested in knowing this hormone when we tell you that it also regulates how you look. This is because estrogen influences fat deposition in your body and skin health as well. Disturbance in the levels of estrogen in your body can lead to a large number of problems such as irregular or absent periods, painful and heavy menstruation, hot flashes, mood swings, sleep disturbance, lethargy, sudden weight changes, breast tenderness or lumpy breasts and vaginal dryness.

HOW DO HORMONES CHANGE WITH AGE AND TIME?

As a woman moves through the different phases of her lifecycle, her hormones also go through significant changes which affects her body functions. Aging means that hormone levels begin to change, some might increase and some might decrease. Whether it be onset of puberty, pregnancy, or menopause, every phase of your life affects the functioning of your hormones as well.

The changes in the levels of female hormones begin when you are as young as 8 years old. Although the average age for the onset of puberty is 11, but it is highly likely that girls may develop breasts and pubic hair and start menstruation before they reach the eleventh year of their life.

As you reach puberty, it takes your body time to adjust to hormonal changes and the levels of hormones begin to rise and stabilize gradually which can often result in irregular menstruation. It takes your body about 4 years to adjust to the hormonal changes that occur at the onset of puberty. Other hormone-related problems which can arise during this phase include acne, mood swings, weight changes, and complications like endometriosis which is the development of uterine muscle outside of the uterus.

The hormonal changes that occur during puberty also influence your sexual behavior. Girls become more interested in sex at this age and begin to feel more attracted towards men and the appeal for sexual pleasure increases. This might also lead you to the concept of birth control and safer ways of having sex. Using birth control introduces hormones into you body from external sources which can prove to be a double-edges sword. As it diminishes some hormonal functions, it may trigger other hormonal complications as well.

As you mature and reach the age of 40-45 years, your hormone levels naturally begin to decrease. Your body enters the phase of perimenopause. Until this phase you have a normal menstrual cycle and from this time onwards, you might experience irregular menstruation and other symptoms like night sweats, hot flushes, and mood swings. The time for a woman to reach perimenopause phase varies but usually begins after a woman reaches her forties.

When you reach the age above 45, the levels of estrogen start to drop very rapidly. This results in the stoppage of egg release from ovaries and as a result your no longer have a menstrual cycle and periods. At this age a woman cannot get pregnant naturally. Science says that a woman is said to have reached menopause if she does not have periods for more than a year. The average age for menopause in females is 50-52 years. Menopause is associated with many symptoms due to hormonal changes which include sleep problems, anxiety, and hot flushes. Menopause is usually the last phase of a woman's life where drastic hormonal shifts occur.

2. UNDERSTANDING HORMONE IMBALANCE

Hormone imbalance is the name given to a situation where the level of one or more hormones in your body is either too high or too low than its normal level. Hormones, being the chemical messengers of the body perform very important functions and even a very slight disturbance in their levels can cause many health-related problems. The imbalance of even one hormone can cause havoc in your body as it affects the functioning of other organs and glands as well which start to work extraordinarily to cover the complications caused by this imbalance.

As life is advancing day by day, hormone imbalance is also become very common in both men and women. However, women fall prey to hormonal imbalance more rapidly and severely due to their complex system of hormones that regulates the menstrual cycle and pregnancy.

As your age progresses, the levels of hormones continue to shift due to your changing physiology but hormone imbalance refers to an abnormal change in the normal levels of hormones which is caused by some external factor or disease.

WHY DO HORMONES LOSE BALANCE?

Hormone imbalance can occur as a result of a large number of factors of varying nature. Sometimes hormone imbalance can occur due to natural causes like menopause, breastfeeding and pregnancy. In other cases, hormone imbalance can result from an underlying disease like diabetes, cancer or some genetic disorders or cardiovascular diseases. Other culprits of hormone imbalance include stress, trauma or injury, or use of certain medications (birth control pills). Let's have a detailed insight into the main causes of hormone imbalance and the mechanism behind it.

1. **Stress**

Unfortunately, stress is a stranger to no one. Every woman is likely to feel stressed in her life at one point or another. In fact, the modern and sedentary lifestyles which we have adopted over time are triggers for stress and as a result hormonal imbalance.

Being stressed on occasions for a short period of time is normal. However, staying in a stressed state of mind of extended periods of time can be detrimental to your hormones. This is because naturally your body produces some stress hormones i.e., adrenaline and cortisol which help manage your body's response to a stressful situation. Staying under stress for prolonged periods can increase the levels of these hormones in the blood stream to an extent where they cause imbalance, start affecting the functioning of other hormones and cause symptoms like insomnia, irregular menstruation, obesity, fertility issues and reduced libido.

2. Trauma

Trauma is very closely-related to stress. You must be fully aware that any kind of trauma can disturb your mental health but you should also know that trauma can also cause physical disturbance in your body include hormonal imbalance.

When you undergo any kind of trauma like childhood abuse, death of a loved one, or a car accident then your body activates its stress response system because trauma is actually being in a constant state of stress. This stress response is a good thing as it is your body's natural way of coping with traumatic situations. However, if trauma lasts for a long period of time that it can dysregulate the hypothalamic-pituitary-adrenal (HPA) axis which is the stress response system of your central nervous system. This causes an imbalance of hormones which are managed by the hypothalamus, pituitary and adrenal glands.

Cortisol and oxytocin are the main hormones affected by trauma. You must have gotten quite familiar with cortisol by now as we mentioned previously that it is the stress hormone. Oxytocin is the love hormone of your body. Its release is affected by trauma and low levels of oxytocin can cause decreased sociability and sex drive.

3. Brain injury

Brain injury can damage the two main glands of your body i.e., the hypothalamus and the pituitary gland. This can result in a large number of hormonal imbalances. A hormone may be released too less and another may be released too much. This can totally disrupt your body's homeostasis i.e., stability of internal biological environment including balance of fluids, salt, water, blood pressure and body temperature. Hormonal imbalance due to brain injury can cause symptoms like depression, sexual dysfunction, headaches, gastrointestinal disturbance, mood swings, irregular menstruation and weight changes.

4. Menopause

Menopause is a natural phenomenon that occurs in every woman's life when she reaches the age of 45-55. A large number of hormonal changes occur when you reach the perimenopause or menopause phase of your life. The levels of female sex hormones like estrogen, progesterone and testosterone are totally changed during this time which results in a large number of symptoms and physical changes. Estrogen production is reduced to a very low-level during menopause which results in symptoms like hot flashes, night sweat, insomnia, fatigue, palpitations and breast tenderness. Progesterone levels also start to fall as you reach perimenopause. During this time, the last periods become very heavy, irregular, painful and longer. Therefore, menopause is associated with many hormonal changes and imbalances which cause a large number of physical symptoms.

5. Pregnancy

Pregnancy is probably the most dramatic hormonal event that can occur in your life. It results in a large number of physiological changes in your body which include both your physical health and hormonal health. As you become pregnant, there is a sudden and dramatic rise in the level of estrogen and progesterone in your body. There isn't a change in the levels of estrogen and progesterone alone. Many other hormones also undergo imbalances during this time.

The levels of estrogen rise in order to stimulate the uterus to support the fetus and development of placement for the transfer of nutrients from mother to fetus and enhancement of blood circulation. Progesterone levels also become unusually high during pregnancy. This change occurs in order to stimulate the internal organs like uterus to increase in size for the growth of fetus. It also relaxes ligament and joints during pregnancy.

6.   Breastfeeding

There is a lot happening with your hormones during and post-pregnancy. One of the processes that causes immense hormonal fluctuations is breastfeeding. After delivering the baby and the placenta, the estrogen levels in your body begin to decline. This triggers the production of the milk-producing hormone i.e., prolactin. This has a significant impact on vaginal tissue and results in decrease in vaginal flexibility and thickness of vaginal wall. It also causes irritation and dryness in the vagina which results in painful intercourse and burning while urination.

7.   Medications

Some medications especially birth control pills can cause havoc in your hormonal system. Birth control pills contain synthetic hormones. Normally, the natural estrogen and progesterone formed in your body bind to very particular receptors that are specific to these hormones only. However, taking synthetic progesterone in the form of birth control pills can through your body off balance. This is because synthetic hormones can bind to other receptors as well which can send inaccurate signals to your brain causing unwanted physiological responses that can lead to a lot of hormonal problems. They can interfere with the functioning of normal flora in your microbiome and cause gut problems. They can sometimes also result in depletion of essential micronutrients.

8. **Underlying diseases**

Diabetes

Diabetes and hormonal imbalance are linked both ways. Usually, diabetes develops as a result of hormone imbalance. When your body develops a resistance to insulin in your body and the blood sugar levels begin to rise, the pancreas works hard to produce more insulin but it can't keep up with the rising insulin resistance. As a result, high blood levels of glucose lead to type II diabetes. However, diabetes also causes further hormone imbalances in your body.

If you are in your menopause then you are likely to experience much worse symptoms of hormone imbalance if you also have diabetes. Your libido decreases and damage to vaginal tissue occurs due to low level of hormones. This also results in a lot of pain during intercourse. It can result in sleep disturbance and increased incidence of hot flashes and night sweats.

Cancer

Cancer is one of the most problematic causes when it comes to hormone imbalance due to underlying diseases. The levels of your hormones can be thrown completely off balance if you have cancer or are getting some kind of cancer treatment. Some cancer cells also produce excessive hormones which cause many physical symptoms. Sometimes cancer treatments can lower the levels of certain hormones in your body or even block the production of a particular hormone altogether. Such hormonal imbalances as result of cancer treatment can be temporary or even permanent.

Cancers of the breast, uterus, ovary, and cervix are the leading causes of hormonal imbalance due to cancer. They interfere with the levels of sex hormones and cause a large number of symptoms.

Genetic disorders

Hormonal imbalance is more likely to be caused by any of the conditions mentioned above and rarely it could be genetic. But people who have a genetic history of problems or conditions that cause symptoms of hormone imbalance are at a greater risk of developing those conditions as well.

There are some inherited diseases or genetic abnormalities which can cause an imbalance of endocrine hormones as well. Such diseases include the following:

- Multiple endocrine neoplasia 1, 2, and 3 which affects multiple endocrine glands (hypothalamus, pituitary, adrenal and thyroid) causing an imbalance of their hormones.

- Phaeochromocytoma is a rare genetic disorder which causes formation of tumors around the adrenal glands leading to abnormality in functioning of adrenal hormones like adrenaline and cortisol which dysregulates the stress response system of your body.

- Congenital adrenal hyperplasia is an inherited disorder of the adrenal glands whereby adrenal glands produce abnormal hormones which interfere with the normal functioning of immune system and disturb the blood pressure, stress responses and metabolism of your body.

SIGNS AND SYMPTOMS OF HORMONE IMBALANCE

As your body contains more than 50 different hormones each having its own function to control a particular process in your body, you are very likely to experience varying symptoms of hormone imbalance depending on the hormone which is affected. However, it is very important to keep track of what you are feeling and if you notice any change in your mental or physical health which is affecting your normal bodily functions or your overall health in general.

Every woman has a different body and it is possible that you may experience a symptom of imbalance in a particular hormone and another woman having the same imbalance may not experience that symptom. Therefore, you always need to check with your physician when you experience any unusual symptom in your body which could point to hormone imbalance or any other problem.

Here is a list of all the symptoms of hormone imbalance that can possibly occur as a result of imbalance in your metabolic hormones, stress hormones, sex hormones or any other type of hormones:

Reproductive symptoms

- Irregular or absent menstruation
- Heavy periods
- Difficulty in conceiving or reduced fertility
- Reduced sex desire

Physical symptoms

- Intense abdominal cramps
- Hirsutism
- Fatigue
- Hair fall
- Hot flashes
- Night sweats
- Numbness in hands and feet or fingers and toes
- Feeling too hot or too cold
- Sweaty palms
- Brittle bones
- Blurred vision
- Irregular heartbeat
- Higher level of cholesterol in blood
- Painful and frequent urination

- Breast tenderness
- Insomnia or difficulty sleeping
- Dryness of hair
- Increased thirst
- Headaches

Skin-related symptoms

- Acne on face and back
- Itchy and dry vagina
- Growth of tiny clusters of skin (skin tags) on your body
- Coarse, rough and dry skin
- Blackening of skin around the base of neck and in armpits
- Skin rashes

Digestive symptoms

- Bloating
- Constipation
- Diarrhea or excessive bowel movement
- Eating disorders

Weight-related symptoms

- Irregular distribution of fat in your body
- Sudden loss or gain of weight
- Difficulty losing weight

Nervous symptoms

- Irritability
- Anxiety
- Depression
- Mood swings

IMPACT OF HORMONE IMBALANCE ON FEMALE REPRODUCTIVE HEALTH

When talking about hormone imbalance in females the first thing that comes to mind is problems in menstruation and reproduction. The female reproductive system is entirely governed by hormone balance and a slight disturbance in the level of a hormone greatly affects your reproductive health. We can fit the impact of hormone imbalance on female reproductive health in three major categories:

1. **Period-related problems**

The most common symptom of hormone imbalance seen in women is irregular period. An irregular period is when the time between two periods is either less than 24 days or more than 38 days. Also, if the length of your cycle varies each month by more than 20 days then such a situation is also termed as irregular periods. The presence of irregular period is considered normal if you are just in your early 2-3 years of menstruation or are reach menopause. But other than that, irregular periods are linked to hormonal imbalance.

An imbalance in the levels of estrogen and progesterone hormones is the greatest cause of period-related problems in females. The Impact of hormone imbalance on your period cycle is not just limited to irregular periods it can also cause your periods to become completely absent or be very heavy and painful.

2. Fertility problems

If you have been trying to get pregnant for more than a year but are unsuccessful than a major cause could be hormone imbalance. The probability of getting pregnant within a year of unprotected sex is more than 84%. So, if you are unable to get pregnant than there could likely be an issue with your hormones.

An irregular period is among the main causes of infertility. if your period occurs too often for example after 2 or 3 weeks than it becomes hard for your uterus to implant and protect a fertilized egg as it doesn't get enough time to sustain the fertilized egg and in turn its lining begins to shed causing another period. And if your period occurs after more than 40-50 days then it means your ovaries are not releasing enough eggs for fertilization which in turn makes pregnancy difficult. All of this is related to hormone imbalance which is the leading cause behind period related problems as discussed previously.

3. Disturbance in menstrual cycle during various phases of life

Hormonal imbalance can affect your reproductive or menstrual cycle during various phases of your life. It can affect the onset of puberty, cause irregular periods during teenage or cause period-related issued during menopause.

The onset of puberty or start of periods in a girl usually occurs any time between the age of 10-16 years. If you or any other girl you know did not get her period during this age then there is a probability of hormonal imbalance. A girl is likely to have onset of periods around the same time as her mother. Hormonal imbalance due to weight changes or dietary problems or other environment factors can cause this issue.

Early teens and late teens also undergo hormonal imbalance sometimes when their reproductive system is still in development or maturation phase. This causes irregular periods because their hormonal system is not totally developed which is why their cycle undergoes irregular changes.

Entering menopause which is also called the perimenopause phase is also associated with irregular menstruation and a lot of hormonal changes. This usually occurs when you reach your late 40s. your periods may skip, be very frequent or sometimes can be unusually heavier or lighter. Such hormonal imbalance during menopause is often faced by a large percentage of women.

MOST COMMON HORMONAL IMBALANCES FACED BY WOMEN

Your body's normal physiology is regulated by your hormonal system. A slight imbalance of hormones can result in a large number of problems in your body which can affect almost every biological system. Let's have a look at the most common type of hormone imbalances women face and how they affect their health:

1.   **Poly cystic ovarian syndrome (PCOS)**

Research has shown that approximately 6-12% of women suffer from PCOS while they are in the reproductive age of their life. PCOS occurs when there is an imbalance of testosterone in your body. This imbalance hinders the release of eggs from ovaries. Instead, small cysts begin to form in your ovaries which result in further hormone imbalances and period-related problems.

The most common symptoms of PCOS include weight gain, acne, hirsutism, irregular or absent periods and difficulty in losing weight. PCOS is also a great risk factor for type 2 diabetes as the hormone imbalance disrupts blood sugar levels and increases insulin resistance in your body.

2. **Thyroid disorders**

Disturbance in thyroid hormones can result in either of the two conditions i.e., hyperthyroidism of hypothyroidism. Hyperthyroidism is the name given to an overactive thyroid gland where it produces too much thyroid hormones which can cause symptoms like weight loss and extremely high energy levels. Hypothyroidism is the name given to an underactive thyroid where it produces very less thyroid hormones which can cause symptoms like weight gain and too low energy levels.

Any of the two thyroid disorders can result in period related problems. It can cause your periods to become irregular, very heavy, painful or even absent for a few months. Thyroid problems may occur as a result of a genetic problem, cancer, or any other underlying disease.

3. **Estrogen imbalances**

Estrogen imbalances are most common in women who are nearing menopause or have reached menopause. Estrogen imbalance can occur due to a variety causes ranging from trauma, injury, stress, birth control, or menopause in general.

The presence of too little estrogen in your body can cause your periods to be very light or completely absent. This is also very common in women with very low body fat such as those with eating disorders or athletes.

The presence of too much estrogen in your body can cause your period to become very heavy, lengthy and painful. This is usually common in women who have excess body fat. Estrogen imbalances are associated with other symptoms like mood swings, fatigue, headache, pain during intercourse hot flashes and breast tenderness.

4.   Progesterone imbalances

Progesterone is the one of the most important sex hormones in females that is released by ovaries and is very important for pregnancy. Progesterone imbalances are very common in women and can result from a poor diet, sedentary lifestyle, stress, pregnancy, trauma, injury and use of birth control. Progesterone imbalances are associated with symptoms like low sex drive, infertility, and depression.

5.   Prolactin imbalances

Prolactin is the hormone produced by your pituitary gland which is important during pregnancy and breast feeding. Prolactin imbalances can occur due to genetic pituitary disorders, cancer of the pituitary gland and certain liver diseases. Symptoms of prolactin imbalance include unusual discharge from your nipples even when you are not pregnant, swollen and tender breasts, fertility problems, fatigue and headaches.

3. MANAGING HORMONE IMBALANCE

The hormone regulation system of your body has a significant affect on how your body performs mentally, physically and emotionally. This means that your hormones have a big say in controlling your moods, emotions, reproductive health and weight. What you eat and how you spend your day in terms of physical activity greatly impacts your hormone balance. Every hormone is secreted in a precise amount in your body, each having its own specific functions. A little imbalance in their levels can have a negative affect on your health and cause serious complications in the long term. A sedentary lifestyle coupled with an unhealthy diet can be disastrous for your hormone balance. The first step to managing hormone balance is a change in your lifestyle by adoption of healthy eating habits and good physical activity. In the next page you are going to discover are some diet and lifestyle changes which you can adopt to bring your imbalance hormone cycle back on track.

DIET TIPS

Consume more proteins

Protein is a vital component of your nutrient requirements. They are the building blocks from which most of the hormones are made up of. Consuming more protein can greatly help in reviving your hormones back to their healthy state. Amino acids (components of proteins) are the essential nutrients which your body cannot produce on its own and their need must be met by diet.

Hormones made from proteins (peptide hormones) are required for managing a large number of physiological processes such as metabolism, growth, stress management, reproduction, and appetite. The amount of protein you intake directly influences your hormonal functioning and impacts the energy consumption system of your body.

Science has proven that proteins have the ability to make you feel full, lessen your food cravings and result in weight loss due to less food intake. This is because proteins reduce the activity of your hunger hormone i.e., ghrelin and stimulate the hormones that make you feel fuller i.e., Glucagon-Like Peptide-1. Therefore, consuming more proteins is the first step you can take towards managing your hormonal disturbances.

The choice of proteins you intake also has a great say in your body's nutritional requirements. Both animal and plant proteins should be consumed in moderate amounts. It is essential that you consume organic, fresh and healthy farm-based, grass-fed meat and not unhealthy, steroid-fed factory-farmed meat.

Some of the best sources of protein include eggs, milk, lean meat, chicken, lentils, and fish like salmon. Plant-based protein sources include spinach, artichokes, sweet potatoes, Brussels spouts and broccoli.

Consume healthy fats

Good fats are a driving force for hormones. They require healthy fats and cholesterol to carry out their normal functions and even some hormones (lipid-based hormones) are made up of fats. Furthermore, inclusion of healthy fats in your daily diet can help reduce insulin resistance associated with hormonal problems like PCOS. It reduces your appetite and prevents overeating.

One kind of healthy fats are medium-chain triglycerides. These are very unique type of fats which when enter the body, are not stored as excess fat rather immediately used up by the liver to produce energy thus, improving the calorie-burning capacity of your body and enhancing weight loss.

Omega-3 fatty acids are also very essential nutrients that come under the category of healthy fats. They reduce inflammation and stress in the body by alleviating the levels of cortisol which is the stress hormone. Any hormonal imbalances can be managed very well by consuming omega-3s from healthy sources like fatty fish.

The best sources of healthy fats include coconut oil, egg yolk, avocados, olives, almonds, and nuts like peanuts and macadamia. Ghee or butter delivery from grass-fed dairy also nutritious sources of healthy fats. Fish oil and cod liver oil can be very beneficial when consumed in calculated amounts as they improve digestion, cardiac health, metabolism and impart a feeling of fullness.

Consume more fibers

Fibers are the best gut-friendly food that you can consume. It helps improve digestion and stimulates your body's sensitivity to insulin thus maintaining moderate sugar levels and reducing symptoms of PCOS. Fibers stimulate the production of hormones that make you feel full thus reducing your appetite and aiding in weight loss.

The levels of estrogen which is the main hormone of female reproductive system are greatly dependent on your fiber intake. If you do not consume enough fibers then your digestive system will not work properly due to which excess estrogen will not be excreted leading to a problem called estrogen dominance. This can result in numerous unwanted problems like bloating, cramping, breast tenderness, irregular menstruation, decreased sex drives, mood swings, sleep disturbances and anxiety. This is why consumption of healthy levels of fibers is very important to maintain hormonal balance in your body.

Every woman, irrespective of her age should consume at least 20-25g of fiber every day. You should add some fiber in every meal of the day to maintain a good balance of hormones in your body.

There is no need to worry about. Fibers are easily found in your everyday dietary items such as whole grains (brown rice, wheat flour), seeds (flax, chia, pumpkin, sesame), fruits (grapefruit, mango, apple, berries, oranges), beans (kidney, black, garbanzo), nuts (hazelnuts, peanuts, cashews, almonds) and certain vegetables (carrots and beetroot).

Decrease sugar intake

If you have hormone imbalance then sugar is your enemy. This sneaky dietary item is a silent disruptor of your hormone balance. You may think of sugar as only a stimulant for weight gain but this is not just the only way sugar affects your body. The problematic effects of sugar go way beyond just a threat to your waistline. It can mess with the levels of your insulin hormone and result in serious medical conditions like hormonal problems (PCOS), diabetes, obesity and heart issues.

Sugar intake does not include just the sweet stuff like candies, chocolates and desserts. It also includes all the carbohydrate items which are made up of sugars such as potatoes. Yes, my friend, the fries you love are not good for your hormones.

PCOS is a very common hormonal problem in women and it is greatly affected by how much sugar you give to your body on a daily basis. High intake of sugar enhances the insulin resistance of muscular and fatty cells in your body which can lead to an imbalance of the reproductive hormone, estrogen. Even if you don't have PCOS, then excessive sugar intake can cause symptoms of hormonal imbalance like mood swings, irritability, sleep disturbances, anxiety and depression.

Despite all the haunting implications of a high sugar diet, you don't need to worry. Everything you eat or feed your body is always under your control. All you have to do is start with simple steps and cut down you daily sugar intake slowly. If you take 2 spoons of sugar in your morning coffee cup then reduce it to one. Use healthy alternatives like organic and natural honey which can fulfil your sweet cravings without harming your hormone balance.

Quit alcohol intake

Among the many things that can throw off the balance of your hormones, alcohol is one of the toppers. This popular comfort drink does not just make your brain go woozy but it can also whack your hormonal system in a very problematic way. The issue doesn't lie in very occasional, small amounts of alcohol use rather in chronic cases of alcohol abuse.

Alcohol affects almost every system of your body and the endocrine system is the most affected in this case. Alcohol can affect the following hormones in your body:

- "Feel good" or happy hormones – dopamine, oxytocin and serotonin
- Sugar regulating hormones – insulin and glucagon
- Reproductive hormones – estrogen, progesterone and testosterone
- Stress hormones – cortisol
- Hormones that regular bone health – growth hormone

The ability of alcohol to impact reproductive hormones can greatly affect your fertility in the long run. It also greatly influences oxytocin which is linked to your emotions like love and bonding as result of which it can impact your sexual desires.

Alcohol intake can worsen the symptoms of menopause in older women. They may experience enhanced sleep problems, intense hot flashes and increased anxiety. Alcohol can increase the risk of suffering from diseases like breast cancer and diabetes. It can worsen PMS symptoms and cause greater problems after chronic use.

Although, alcohol abuse can be very dangerous for your hormones but there is always a way of correcting everything. If you are an alcoholic and want to avoid hormonal problems then start working on withdrawing from this bad habit now.

Adopt a Rainbow diet

A rainbow diet is a diet that includes intake of foods that match all colors of the rainbow. The foods mostly include fruits and vegetables. Intake of such a variety of food species in your weekly dietary routine can fulfil all the nutritious requirements of your body and improve your hormonal health as well as immunity.

Rainbow diet involves all the different fruits and vegetables that are rich in minerals and nutrients like iron, magnesium, zinc, omega-3 fatty acids, anti-oxidants, fibers, healthy fats, phytoestrogens and proteins. Some examples of foods you can include in your rainbow diet are as follows:

- Red – apples, cherry, watermelon, strawberry, raspberry, beetroot
- Orange –– orange, sweet potato, pumpkin, peach, apricot
- Yellow –– banana, saffron, yellow bell pepper, corn,
- Green – spinach, broccoli, avocado, cabbage, cauliflower, cucumber, coriander, olive
- Blue – blue berries
- Purple –– plum, brinjal, raisins, black currant, onion, purple cabbage
- White – coconut, mushroom, garlic, radish

LIFESTYLE TIPS

Adapt an active daily routine

One of the biggest drawbacks of today's technological and machine-based world is the sedentary and unhealthy lifestyle that it has rendered to us humans. On an average every person sits for more than 15 hours per day. This constant sitting can result in a large number of health problems including obesity, lethargy, diabetes, and hormonal imbalance. Among the biggest victims of a sedentary lifestyle is your hormone regulation system. The growth hormones are most affected by such an inactive daily routine. This hinders your body's ability to rebuild itself and grow from the damages of stress and anxiety of everyday life. High levels of stress can worsen your hormonal imbalance symptoms like mood swings, irritability, and sleep disturbances.

Therefore, the first step in managing hormonal imbalance is getting active. Try increasing your daily step count by taking walking breaks almost every hour while at work. If you do a home-based or online job where you have to sit in front of a desk or computer all the time, then you should schedule your routine in a way to fit at least an hour of exercise or workout so that you can compensate for all the inactive and sitting time. Make small changes like using the stairs instead of the elevator. Try walking to work or for grocery runs. Incorporate small exercises and stretching while doing minimal at-home tasks like watching TV. These slight changes may feel minimal but they can make a big difference and greatly help in managing your hormone imbalance.

Maintain a moderate weight

Obesity is one of the greatest enemies of your hormones. Your broad waistline is not just a problem for your looks but also a big issue for your hormone regulation system. Being overweight can greatly affect the insulin sensitivity of your body and in turn lead to complicated hormonal problems.

Insulin resistance is enhanced in the body of a person who is overweight which can result in problems like Type II diabetes and cardiovascular diseases. Obese women are also vulnerable to disturbance in levels of reproductive hormones because obesity reduce the production of hormones from ovaries which can lead to infertility and problems like PCOS. This means that maintaining a moderate and healthy weight is essential when it comes to managing hormone imbalance.

You can lose weight by making dietary changes in your every day life. Try to cut down sugars and processed foods from your diet. Avoid intake of fast food like pizza, burgers and fries. Carbonated drinks are very high in sugar content which is the main culprit behind obesity. Replace your intake of carbonated drinks with fresh fruit juices and smoothies.

A healthy diet for losing weight works best in combination with exercise. Take some time out from your everyday routine and fit in daily walk and exercise. Try stretching, yoga and interesting ways of losing weight like dancing, aerobics. Make your hormone balancing journey fun and interesting rather than thinking of it as a burden.

Ensure good gut health

Your gut is the busiest system of your body as it contains trillions of bacteria which regulate your hormonal functions in one way or the other. These bacteria are responsible for producing different metabolites which can affect your hormone health either in a positive or negative way.

The microbiome of your gut helps regulate your hormonal functions by affecting the feelings of fullness and insulin sensitivity in your body. Fibers are the best friends of your gut. When fibers are fermented by bacteria in your gut, they produce healthy fatty acids like acetates which work to reduce insulin resistance in your body by increase your body's ability to burn calories. These substances also promote a feeling of fullness and prevent you from overeating and gaining more weight which is itself a great risk factor for hormone imbalance as discussed above. This means that it is very important that you keep you gut in a healthy state so that the microbiome can work positively.

The best way to ensure good gut health is to consume more fibers. The foods that are rich in fibers include whole grains (brown rice, wheat flour), seeds (flax, chia, pumpkin, sesame), fruits (grapefruit, mango, apple, berries, oranges), beans (kidney, black, garbanzo), nuts (hazelnuts, peanuts, cashews, almonds) and certain vegetables (carrots and beetroot). Taking probiotic supplements can also greatly help restore the good bacteria in your gut thus leading to maintenance of hormone balance.

Ensure a healthy sleep cycle

No matter how healthy you eat or how active you are every day, as long as you don't get enough good-quality sleep every day, nothing in your body can function properly. A poor sleep routine can lead to disturbance in levels of a large number of hormones including insulin, ghrelin, cortisol and growth hormone.

The relationship between hormones and sleep is like a two-way street. Disturbance of one causes problem in the other. Consistent lack of a good night's sleep can poorly influence your hormone levels and lead to problems like irregular menstruation, obesity, adrenal problems, and diabetes. Therefore, getting at least 8 hours of a consistent and peaceful sleep is essential to maintain hormone balance stay healthy overall.

Here are some ways you can improve your sleep routine:

- Set up a bed time every day and be consistent with it. Make sure to complete all your tasks before bed time.
- Reduce the brightness of your smart phones and electronic devices. The blue light from smartphones disturbs your sleep cycle by unbalancing the sleep hormone, melatonin.
- Ensure good water intake throughout the day.
- Keep your mind stress-free.
- Try reading a light and fun book to bed so that your mind becomes stress-free. In this way you can sleep peacefully.
- Always ensure to sleep in a dark and quiet room. Noise and light can disrupt your brain and stimulate your senses which can cause you to wake up frequently.

Reduce stress levels

Stress is very strongly linked to your hormonal endocrine system. It is the biggest enemy of your hormone happiness. When your body is in a state of stress, the level of your stress hormone i.e., cortisol is increased. This can compromise the functioning of all the systems of your body as cortisol dominance can consume all the body's energy for managing stress. This also indirectly affects all the other hormones which are in turn put to the backburner.

Such a stressful condition for your body has a very negative impact on your reproductive hormones as well. High levels of cholesterol lead to lesser production of progesterone during the ovulatory and luteal phase of menstrual cycle which can result in high levels of estrogen in response. This can result in estrogen dominance which is linked to serious hormonal complications like PCOS, worsening of menopause symptoms and even infertility. Therefore, it is very important to keep your body stress-free in order to ensure good hormonal balance.

Try to manage your stress level by adopting the following ways:

- Spend at least 30 minutes to one hour in nature every day. Nature is so peaceful and refreshing that it can help relax your mind and alleviate stress and anxiety levels. This is not just a myth its actually proven by science.
- Ensure a good sleep routine of 8 hours every day. A stress-free mind is a rested mind. Sleep helps relax your nerves and gives your brain some time to heal.
- Ensure a good balance between your work and personal life. Do not overstrain yourself with anything that messes with your mental health. Set boundaries for everything and do not compromise on your mental peace.
- Be more social with your friends and family members. Try to share and convey your problems. Talking and sharing greatly helps in freeing your mind from the stress and improves your mood.

Quit smoking

Smoking, irrespective of it being active or passive, can wreak havoc in your body. It is a silent killer that can influence your hormones in every negative way possible. Smoking has a very bad influence on all kinds of hormones. The most affected are reproductive hormones i.e., estrogen, progesterone and testosterone. Smoking reduces the levels of estrogen in your body when it is mostly needed. This can mess with your reproductive cycle and also influences the onset of menopause.

Another very problematic impact of smoking is the ability of nicotine toxins to affect the anti-Mullerian hormone which is responsible for protecting the reserve of eggs in your ovaries. Smoking reduces the levels of this hormone and thus endangers the safety of eggs in ovarian follicles which can directly lead to fertility problems.

The prolactin hormone, which is responsible for milk production in breast-feeding women, is also affected in chain smokers. The toxic components of cigarette smoke reduce levels of prolactin in the body thus reducing milk production after pregnancy.

Smoking also worsens symptoms of hormone imbalance like irregular menstruation, painful periods, cramps, insomnia, mood swings and hot flashes during menopause.

Although quitting smoking is not an easy task but it is very important if you want to manage your hormone levels.

Here are some small and minimal tips which can help you in your journey of quitting smoking towards a better hormonal future:

- List your goals and reasons for quitting.
- Share your goals with your friends and family so they can encourage you.
- Try using stop smoking aids after consultation with your doctor.
- Keep yourself busy.
- Try to divert your mind when you are craving a smoke.
- List what triggers your cravings and make efforts to avoid them.
- Join therapy groups and socialize with people who have quit before or are in the process of quitting to get some tips.

4. NATURAL HERBS AND INGREDIENTS

Natural herbs are not only the best ingredients for cooking but have also proven to be highly beneficial in health care for managing numerous medical conditions. Experiencing healing through natural remedies and organic ways is very satisfying and aesthetically pleasing. Human kind has been using natural herbs for health purposes for thousands of years. Balancing hormones through natural remedies is therapeutic and can help alleviate symptoms of hormonal imbalance. Here are some natural herbs and ingredients which can help keep your hormones in balance:

Black cohosh root

Native to the eastern regions of North America, Black Cohosh root belongs to a white flowering plant, scientifically known as Actaea racemose. This herb may also be known by the name of snakeroot, rattletop or bugbane. Besides its anti-inflammatory action and soothing effects on nervous system, the herb is most commonly known for its beneficial impact on female hormonal health, especially for menopausal women.

Black cohosh is known to act as phytoestrogen (a plant-based substitute of estrogen) in the body. In this way it influences the functioning of estrogen in the body and can reduce menopausal symptoms like hot flashes, sleep disturbances, anxiety and night sweats. It balances the sleep cycle and helps in management of hormone balance by reducing severity of PMS, PMDD, PCOS and other complications of hormonal imbalance.

This wondrous herb can also enhance fertility and help alleviate menstrual irregularities to make pregnancy possible for women suffering from PCOS.

You can buy the root from your local herbalist and incorporate it into your daily routine in the form of an extract or tea. It helps regulate normal functioning of menstrual cycle and improves bone health. Calming and soothing effects on the nervous system are a bonus!

Ashwagandha

Derived from the roots of Withania somnifera, Ashwagandha is a superb herb that has been used in medicine for thousands of years in the Indian Subcontinent. Also known as Indian Ginseng and winter cherry, the herb belongs to the nightshade family and is loaded with the richness of alkaloids and anti-oxidants. These and other anti-inflammatory properties make Ashwagandha a powerful adaptogen. This means that it enhances your body's ability to cope with stress associated with hormonal imbalance.

Ashwagandha is capable of enhancing fertility and reducing the symptoms of PCOS like acne, menstrual irregularities, hirsutism and high levels of blood sugar. This herb can be consumed in the form of an extract, tea, powder, tablet or capsule. You can enhance the benefits of ashwagandha by using it in combination with a high-fiber diet, consuming healthy fats and reducing the intake of processed sugar.

Although menopause may bring about a feeling of freedom in women but it comes with numerous unwanted symptoms. Ashwagandha herbal tea can be extremely beneficial in reducing hot flashes, night sweats, weight gain and bone loss that are the most common symptoms observed in menopausal women.

Chaste tree berry

The secret sauce to your hormonal balance dish is Chaste tree berry. This unpopular berry has abilities of bringing your hormonal cycle back to its normal functioning. Thousands of years of medicinal use are associated with this herb for the purpose of hormone regulation. Scientifically known as Vitex agnus-castus, Chaste tree berry can help regulate the normal physiology of female reproductive cycle.

This natural hormone regulator can treat symptoms of PMS, PCOS, menopause, infertility and other hormonal complications that cause dysregulation of female hormones. It works by balancing the levels of prolactin, elevated levels of which can cause breast pain, and other PMS symptoms.

Also known as Monk's pepper or vitex, this herb has wonderous alleviating properties that will help you go through your pre-menstrual phase smoothly. Breast tenderness, mood swings, migraines, depression, cravings and irritability associated with PMS can be cured with fresh extract of chaste tree berry.

The ability of vitex to regulate levels of prolactin allows this herb to enhance the chances of women to become pregnant. Women facing a difficulty in conceiving can try using this fertility enhancer to remove menstrual irregularities which are the main cause behind infertility, early miscarriages and other pregnancy-related complications.

Nigella seeds

Did you know that the little black seeds you see lying around in your kitchen cabinet can be very helpful for regulating hormonal balance? Nigella seeds or kalonji are produced by the flowers of a plant called Nigella sativa. These seeds are packed with plant based nutrients and have proven to be beneficial in decreasing symptoms of hormonal complications.

Nigella seeds possess estrogen like properties which allow them to normalize female menstrual cycle and decrease unwanted symptoms of menopause. Consuming nigella seeds reduces menstrual irregularities, cramps, smelly discharge and mood swings while you are on your period.

The oil extracted from these seeds has scientifically proven to treat leucorrhea (bad smelling yellowish-white vaginal discharge). If you have this problem then all you have to do is boil some mint leaves in a glass of water. Add 3-4 drops of black seed oil in it after cooling and drink this mixture every day for a month and you will see this problem vanish like it was never there.

Kalonji oil is also very helpful when it comes to preventing uterine cysts and stones. For this purpose, you can take a spoon of honey in a glass of luke warm water, add 3-4 drops of kalonji oil to it and drink it every morning on an empty stomach. This combination works wonders for uterine problems and hormonal imbalance.

Marjoram

Frequently used as a culinary spice in the Mediterranean regions, sweet marjoram belongs to the family of oregano (wild marjoram), thyme and sage. This herb is available in the markets in the form of fresh or dried leaves, extracts and oils.

Owing to its anti-inflammatory and anti-microbial properties, marjoram has numerous health benefits especially for female reproductive health. This wonderous herb is packed with folate which boosts menstrual health and decreases irregularities in female hormonal functioning. A cup of marjoram tea daily can help reduce your cramps during periods and soothe your mental health so that you can pass the 7 days in a care-free way.

Marjoram helps in reducing the severity of PCOS symptoms and is an amazing supplement for managing hormonal imbalance in the most natural and organic ways possible. It helps balance the levels of androgen in the body, relieves unwanted period pains and enhances insulin sensitivity which is often affected during PCOS. It helps restore the problems of a missed period or more than one episode of periods in a single month.

You can incorporate marjoram in your daily routine by adding it in your dishes while cooking, drinking marjoram tea or using it in the form an essential oil.

Dong Quai

As the name suggests, Dong quai is a Chinese herb but is also very popular in the western world of herbal medicine. Belonging to the family of parsley and celery, dong quai or Angelica sinensis has numerous health benefits and has long been used in Chinese herbal medicine for treating female hormone problems.

Also called the 'female ginseng', dong quai root works wonders when it comes to balancing female hormones and reducing symptoms associated with hormonal irregularities. For over 2000 years, dong quai has been used in Japan, China and Korea for its abilities to improve hormone regulation, reduce menstrual complications, relieve menstrual cramps, detoxify blood, enhance immune regulation, and relax bowel movements to reduce stomach problems.

This Chinese angelica root can get rid of toxins from your blood after menstruation and pregnancy. It helps improve the quality of female blood and reduces risk of infections during periods. Dong quai helps in regulating hormonal balance during menopause and reduces unwanted symptoms of menopause like hot flashes, night sweats, and anxiety.

You can also benefit from the wonders of dong quai by drinking tea made by boiling roots of the herb in water and adding a spoon of honey to make it sweet.

Lady's mantle

Owing to the amazing health benefits of this herb, it won't be wrong to call it a woman's best friend. With a history dating back to the medieval times of 1500s, Lady's mantle or Lion's foot, scientifically known as Alchemilla vulgaris, contains tannins and flavonoids which are amazing anti-inflammatory compounds.

The key benefits of this herb revolve around its ability to regulate the menstrual cycle and bring about all hormones to their normal physiology. It enhances progesterone release which is the major hormone behind normal menstrual function. This also improves fertility due to the timely release and implantation of eggs in the uterus. Thus, acting as a tonic for female reproductive system, lady's mantle can surely cure all your hormone related problems.

The tannins present in this herb help reduce excessive bleeding during periods so you want have to use those thick pads and hard cups which is another problem in itself. The herb also curbs menopausal symptoms and reduces the mood swings associated with PMS, PCOS and other phases of the menstrual cycle.

Lady's mantle works for women of all ages whether young or old. It helps improve overall hormone regulation and keeps your body safe from the havoc of hormonal imbalance. The herb can be utilized in the form of a tincture, powder or tea in your daily routine.

Wild Yam

Also called Devil's bones, colic's roots or China root, wild yam is an organic herb traditionally being used in herbal medicine for centuries. Wild yam belongs to the plant Dioscorea villosa L. that is native to northern regions of America and China. It is a vine plant and its roots and bulbs are utilized for their medicinal properties.

This ancient plant can greatly help in managing your hormone imbalance problems. It is surely a boon for women suffering from menstrual cramps and unwanted pains during menopause. The medicinal benefits of wild yam extend to the entire endocrine system. It helps relieve menopausal symptoms like hot flashes and night sweats.

Wild yam contains anti-inflammatory and relaxing compounds called saponins which greatly help in soothing your muscles and reducing inflammation around your abdominal area due to menstrual irregularities.

This wonderous herbal remedy can be consumed along or in combinations with other hormone-balancing herbs like black cohosh. You can prepare a cream, tincture, extract, oil, or tea of the colic root and incorporate it into your daily routine to benefit from the irreplaceable advantages of using this herb.

Kelp

Commonly perceived as a gross and slimy sea green, Kelp has some remarkable health benefits that are surely going to change your perspective about this wonderous sea herb. This culinary king of algae has enriched and packed with numerous minerals, vitamins and hormone-balancing properties that can boost your hormone regulation system and bring a detracted menstrual cycle back on track.

This brown seaweed promotes weight loss, boosts metabolism, reduces blood sugar and inflammation in your body. All these factors impact your hormone balance in one way or the other and this is how kelp can help keep your hormone balance in check. It also reduces levels of thyroid hormone in your body as it contains good amounts of iodine.

Kelp has amazing antibacterial and antifungal properties which helps keep you safe from infections and unwanted hygienic problems. The polyphenols and anti-oxidants present in kelp are very effective in fighting hormone-dependent cancers and other complications linked to hormonal imbalance in women.

You can incorporate this super seaweed in your diet in the form of a green kelp salad or a plate of healthy sushi packed with all those vitamins and minerals you need to keep your hormonal cycles in balance.

Milk thistle

Thanks to hormonal disturbances, menopausal women feel unwanted symptoms like mood swings, irritability, anxiety, tiredness, dry skin and lack of self-esteem. In such a situation, milk thistle can come to your rescue and cause all the excessive hormones in your body to be excreted by way of the liver or gastrointestinal tract leading to a balanced hormonal cycle.

Silymarin is an active ingredient present in milk thistle that is responsible for all the good properties of this herb. This substance also acts as an antioxidant which reduces inflammation and keeps you safe from a large number of diseases ranging from heart problems to liver issues and beyond.

Milk thistle is the ultimate herb every woman needs to boost her overall reproductive health. It provides benefits like increasing production of breast milk, flushing excessive hormones from liver, removing toxins from liver, reducing insulin resistance in PCOS and stimulating liver regeneration.

You can incorporate this beneficial herb in your daily routine by taking 20-30 dops of milk thistle extract in a glass of water every day. The herb is safe to use on a long-term basis and is also effective when consumed in the form of a tea.

Passion flower

Depression is one of the biggest symptoms associated with hormonal imbalance and menopause. Passion flower can be your best friend when it comes to reducing depressive symptoms, night sweats, hot flashes and mood swings during menopause. It also helps treat insomnia and disturbances in your sleep cycle.

Passion flower, scientifically known as Passiflora incarnate, is an all-time-favorite herb that has numerous health benefits for hormone health and overall liver functioning. It detoxifies your body from unwanted substances that can trigger hormonal imbalances. Besides it hormonal benefits, passion flower also enhances quality of sleep and reduces anxiety levels associated with mental disorders.

The stress levels of menopausal women are generally high and passion flower can greatly help to reduce them by enhancing the levels of GABA (γ-Amino Butyric Acid) which is a neurotransmitter responsible for keeping your brain stress-free.

Passionflower can be incorporated in every woman's daily routine in the form of a liquid extract or herbal tea. You can prepare a passion flower tea by boiling a tablespoon each of dried passion flowers and chamomile in a cup of water and adding a teaspoon of honey to sweeten it. Strain your tea and enjoy!

Zizyphus

Native to the warm and subtropical regions of the world, Zizyphus is a shrub or small tree that is known to the world of natural medicine for its varying benefits. It is known for a wide variety of beneficial effects including relief from symptoms of PMS, PCOS and menopause.

Zizyphus helps relieve anxiety, sleep disturbances and muscular pain which you are very likely to experience in menopause, hormonal imbalance or during your period in general. It helps keep the insulin levels of the body in balance which are disturbed by the hormonal irregularities that occur during PCOS.

You can use this herb along with other amazing herbal remedies like Chinese yam, black cohosh and valerian root to benefit from its amazing properties of balancing female hormones.

Coconut oil

Considered to be one of the best natural remedies for hormone balance, coconut oil is packed with nutritious substances that can greatly help you in balancing your hormones and bringing a disturbed menstrual cycle back on track.

Coconut oil is packed with medium-chain fatty acids that enhance your body's metabolic rate thus positively influencing hormonal functions. It keeps your body away from stress by balancing the levels of the most important stress hormone in your body i.e., cortisol. The benefits of coconut oil also extend to your sexual health as it boosts the production of sex hormones like progesterone and estrogen thus keep you in a sound health state.

The antibacterial and antifungal properties of coconut oil help keep female private organs from bacterial and fungal infections which are one of the leading causes of hormonal imbalance for women.

You know that unwanted PCOS symptoms are highly linked to weight gain and obesity. Coconut oil can help you in this domain as well. This occurs due to the ability of coconut oil to enhance the functioning of leptin hormone in your body which is responsible for neutralizing your eating habits thus protecting you from overeating.

There are many ways you can incorporate coconut oil in your daily routine. Making a fresh morning smoothie, a low-calorie coconut cake, scrambled eggs in coconut oil or simply a coconut oil hair or mask is the way to go.

Valerian root

Rooted in the ancient Greek practice of herbal medicine, Valerian root, also known as Valeriana officinalis, is native to some regions of Europe, Asia and North America. The plant has white and pink flowers and its root portion is used in the form of a tea, extract or pills to benefit from its amazing therapeutic actions.

This wonderous herb helps improve your sleep cycle which is quite often disturbed during menopause or hormonal problems like PCOS. This happens because Valerian root enhances the secretion of GABA which is responsible for soothing your mind and making it easier to fall asleep.

The hormonal benefits of valerian root extend towards reducing the symptoms of menopause like anxiety, hot flushes, night sweats and insomnia that can greatly influence your daily routine. Amidst your feminine cycle, the intense menstrual cramps and extreme uterine contractions can be soothed to some extent by consuming a tea made from valerian root.

You can consume valerian root in the form of a tincture, capsule, pill or tea however, pregnant and breast-feeding women should avoid the herb in order to prevent any unwanted side effects.

Motherwort

Belonging to the family of mint, Motherwort is a perennial plant that scientifically goes by the name Leonurus cardiaca. Also known as Lion's tail or throw-wort, this herb can greatly help in reducing symptoms of menopause like hot flushes, night sweats and anxiety. This wonderful herb also acts as a stress reliever and can really boost your mood swings during periods and PMS.

This herb helps regulate your menstrual cycle and can cause that monthly flow to always be on time. The cramps and pain that menstruation brings with it can be lessened by using motherwort as a natural herbal tea.

The calming and relaxing effects of motherwort can greatly help women suffering from amenorrhea caused by stress. As mentioned above the herb is a natural stress reliever so it not only reduces stress and anxiety levels ad thus indirectly improves fertility which could be hampered by an absent period.

If you are suffering from emotional problems like grief, sadness, irritability or anger as a result of hormonal problems then motherwort can really help you in getting rid of all such issues and making you feel better. Thus, your hormonal selfcare needs you to incorporate motherwort in your daily routine as it is not only beneficial for your physical health but emotional health as well.

Dandelion

Dandelion, the dainty white flower you know for its beauty, has numerous health benefits that make it an amazing herbal medicine. As said by Ralph Waldo Emerson, 'a plant whose virtues have yet not been discovered', dandelion is more than just a flower or a weed. It is a highly valued crop in many regions of the world and is known for centuries for its wonderous health benefits.

The plant, scientifically know as Taraxacum officinale, is used in Jordan folk medicine to treat problems like infertility, hormonal imbalance, constipation, liver and kidney disorders, uterine cancer and anorexia.

Dandelion leaves can help reduce estrogen dominance and aid the liver in excreting metabolized estrogens thus eliminating the chance of hormonal problems and even reducing the risk of acquiring cancer due to hormonal disruptions.

There are many ways you can incorporate the dandelion plant in your daily routine. You can prepare a delicious green salad from the fresh raw leaves of the plant. You can use the root to make a herbal tea with a hint of honey to flush all those toxins from your body. You can make healthy smoothies from the roots and leaves in the morning to boost your day with a fresh start.

Maca

Native to the indigenous mountains of Andes, Maca, also known as Peruvian ginseng is being used in traditional medicine for over centuries. Belonging to the same family as broccoli and turnip, maca contains many different minerals and nutrients like amino acids, iron and calcium which render the plant its health benefits.

Maca root has shown to improve overall sexual health and boost your libido. This goes for men as well, as the root has amazing ability of improving the erectile function in men. Women leading to menopause can greatly benefit from the therapeutic actions of this herb. Maca contains nutrients that relieve menopausal discomfort, hot flushes, sleep disturbances and anxiety and help you reach this stage of your life with ease.

This herb has a capability of impacting your overall health and it boost female hormonal regulation therefore leading to a reduction in unwanted side effects associated with hormonal imbalance. These include anxiety, mood swings, menstrual irregularities, acne, sudden weight change, fertility problems and many more.

You can use maca in the form or a powder or tablet. You can add it in your daily morning smoothie or a cereal-based breakfast to enjoy the health-boosting advantages of this herb.

Red raspberry leaf

For being enriched with the amazing benefits of vitamin B, red raspberry leaf has triggered the notion of 'B is the new A+'. The beautiful berries we eat almost everyday are not just the only part of the berry plant that has health benefits. The leaves of red berries are equally advantageous for human health.

Red raspberry leaves are packed with vitamin B. this vitamin is known for its tremendous nutritional value. It helps keep female reproductive health in check and reduces all PMS symptoms like mood swings, irritability and menstrual cramps. It also influences the functioning of estrogen and progesterone positively and keeps these hormones in balance thus reducing the risk of cancer and other complications.

The plant is also useful in the last trimester of pregnancy. It can help reduce nausea and stomach problems, strengthens the uterus for child breath and also stimulates the labor process.

The leaves are enriched with minerals and antioxidants like iron, magnesium, potassium, zinc, and vitamin C, all of which are required for a sound hormonal balance in your body. So next time when you purchase red raspberries, make sure to buy some leaves as well, so you can make that herbal tea you need to keep your hormones in check.

Oat straw extract

Counted among God's good herbs, oat straw comes from the plant known as Avena sativa. Native to Northern America and Northern

Europe, the plan extract is commonly used in traditional medicine for its anti-inflammatory properties. The oats you very commonly eat are the seeds of this plant and the extract is taken from its leaves and stems.

The extract is packed with minerals and nutrients such as iron, magnesium, potassium, phosphorous and zinc, which offer a large number of health benefits like stimulation of hormonal health, brain functional and sexual health.

Traditionally, this extract is also used for its ability to boost your mood and reduce any anxiety, stress or depression associated with hormonal imbalances or problems like PMS, PCOS or menopause. This natural plant extract can balance your hormone-producing glands, strengthen your digestive system and calm your nerves.

This wonderous herb is not just limited to its therapeutic benefits but it poses numerous cosmetic benefits to females as well. The nutrients present in this extract can improve the texture of your hair, make your skin smooth and overall make you look young and bright. So, ladies, what are you waiting for? Go buy some oat straw extract from your local herbalist and make some tea or smoothie now!

Saw Palmetto

Originating from the berries of a small palm tree, saw palmetto has been in medicinal use for centuries. The plant called Serenoa repens, is native to southeastern regions of America and is largely known for its benefits regarding male hormonal health.

Although the plant is largely known for its ability to balance male hormones, prostate levels and prevention of hair loss in men but it has some hidden benefits which favor female hormone balance as well. You all may be familiar with testosterone as a male hormone but it is not just a male hormone. Females also have testosterone in the body which is important for numerous physiological functions. Saw palmetto extract helps keep testosterone in balance in your body and prevent unwanted hormonal issues.

The herbal extract can also reduce hair loss from your scalp and surprisingly induce loss of coarse hair from other regions of your body like face and genitals which is a common side effect associated with hormonal imbalance. The extract can reduce symptoms of menopause like vaginal dryness, sleep disturbances, hot flashes and anxiety.

Saw palmetto can be used in the form of a tincture or extract available from a herbal medicine store and must be used with precaution in pregnant and breastfeeding women.

MINERALS AND NUTRIENTS

When it comes to hormone balance, a diet rich in minerals and nutrients are the key. Here are some micronutrients that are essential for maintaining a health hormonal cycle in your body:

Omega-3 fatty acids

Omega-3 fatty acids are the nutrients which our bodies require for healthy functioning. They cannot be prepared inside the body and thus need to be taken via diet. This nutrient is found in every cell of your body and is very important when it comes to maintaining hormonal balance. They make up the building blocks for production of essential hormones like estrogen and progesterone.

There are no second thoughts on the notion that everything in our body is interlinked. So is inflammation and hormone imbalance. The presence of each contributed to the risk of the other. Omega-3s help reduce inflammation in your body by modulation of its inflammatory response thus indirectly enhancing hormone balance.

Another amazing advantage of Omega-3s is that they balance the levels of blood sugar in your body which are directly linked to insulin resistance, a risk factor of hormone imbalance. It influences the balance of stress hormones and sex hormones.

You can take omega-3 fatty acids in your diet by consuming oily fish. Other sources of these nutrients include nuts and seeds like walnuts, chia seeds and flax seeds.

Vitamin D

A hormone for hormones? This notion is correct when it comes to treating hormonal imbalance with vitamin D. Vitamin D is itself a hormone produced by kidneys that is highly essential for overall female health. Besides its own beneficial functions, this vitamin influences the presence or absence of other minerals such as calcium as well which further emphasize its importance.

Women are very likely to suffer from a deficiency of vitamin D which can cause a disturbance in the levels of estrogen in your body ultimately leading to hormone imbalance and other complications. This leads to unwanted symptoms like weight gain, anxiety, mood swings, hot flashes, and insomnia.

Vitamin D is also essential for the absorption of calcium in your body, both of which are required for good bone health. Absence of both nutrients can cause brittle bones in women leading to early osteoporosis.

Naturally, vitamin D can be consumed by eating fish and meat and drinking milk. The vitamin is also abundantly present in sunlight and sitting in the sun for 30 mins each day can greatly help you.

Probiotics

Although probiotics are mostly known for their digestive benefits, but do you know that they are very valuable when it comes to women's health as well? Probiotics are supplements composed of living microbes that are beneficial for us. In addition to their benefits in promoting digestion, preventing lactose intolerance and treating eczema, probiotics can greatly help in managing hormone imbalance as well.

Probiotics containing the microbe estrobolome can regulate estrogenic functions in a woman's body which can help in preventing conditions associated with estrogen imbalance in the body. These include obesity, cancer, PCOS, infertility, endometriosis and heart problems.

Another major advantage of probiotics is that they can help prevent vaginal yeast infections in women. Scientifically called vaginal candidiasis, this infection can cause problematic symptoms like itchiness, painful urination, smelly discharge, and pain during sexual intercourse. Probiotics for women health contain bacteria that are friendly to vaginal environment and help keep your genitals free from such unwanted infectious guests.

Probiotic supplements are easily available at pharmacies but should only be taken after proper consultation from a professional healthcare provider.

Magnesium

This 12th element of the periodic table is involved in thousands of reactions and processes in the human body. Among these numerous roles of magnesium, the most prominent are hormone balance, reduction of PMS symptoms, muscle relaxation, stabilizing blood sugar levels, preventing migraines and soothing anxiety.

Magnesium is known to improve the levels of progesterone in your body which is the hormone responsible for ovulation. So healthy ovulation can occur when adequate amounts of magnesium are present in your body.

This super mineral also helps in managing and regulating estrogen metabolism in females. It helps keep estrogen levels stable and presents any complications arising from high levels of estrogen in your body. Due to its ability to soothe tightened muscles, magnesium can greatly help in alleviating menstrual cramps.

Magnesium also works for hormone balance by managing the levels of serotonin in your body which is the chemical regulating our mood. Magnesium boosts serotonin and helps keep us in a good mood.

You can incorporate magnesium in your daily routine by consuming whole grains and green leafy vegetables. The mineral can also be found in dried beans and nuts, as well as in yoghurt and low-fat milk.

B vitamins

The family of B vitamins is very nutritious when it comes to managing hormone balance in your body. This group of vitamins include vitamin B1, B3, B6, and B12. All these vitamins have their own beneficial roles each of which helps in hormone regulation in one way or another.

The presence of sufficient levels of vitamin B1 in your body can help regulate your metabolism and prevent symptoms like menstrual cramps, anxiety, fatigue, and painful episodes associated with PMS and menopause.

Also known as niacin, vitamin B3 plays a crucial role in maintain good liver and glandular health. It helps regulate hormonal secretions from the liver and other glands in your body and keeps your system on track.

Vitamin B6 is known for its ability to alleviate painful and problematic menstrual symptoms like cramps, mood swings, irritability, and depression. Cobalamin or vitamin B12 is the most popular vitamin of this family and plays many different roles in your body. It helps regulate the levels of substances like serotonin, dopamine and melatonin which are responsible for regulating our mood, emotions and sleep cycle respectively. It also helps improve nervous function and promotes the production of healthy blood cells thus preventing anemia which is a common problem in menstruating females.

You can take these vitamins as supplements or find them in food sources like meat, dairy products, seafood, green leafy vegetables and legumes.

5. FOODS TO AVOID

The balance of hormones in your body is very sensitive and is affected by a slight change in your dietary patterns or daily routine. Indeed, food is the way to a human's heart, but this notion also goes for the fact that the food you eat can make or break the way your body's physiology works. The way to a healthy life or one full of health problems, both go through the road of food and it's better to avoid the problematic one if you want to lead a sound life. Hormones being the highly important chemical messengers of your body are greatly affected by the food you eat. As discussed in the previous chapters there are many herbal ingredients and natural ways of managing hormonal imbalance, but it is always very important to be aware of foods that can offset your balance of hormones and cause a havoc in your system. So, here's a list of the foods you need to avoid if you are suffering from hormonal imbalance or if you want to avoid this problem in future:

Red meat

Who doesn't love a beautiful grilled beef steak? Umm, probably your general microbiome and specifically the hormone regulation system of your body. In fact, red meat is one of the most harmful and problematic foods you can eat. Red meat is packed with unsaturated fats, also called

Low-Density Lipoproteins (LDLs) or bad cholesterol. These substances are highly dangerous for your body. These LDLs accumulate in your blood vessels and block normal blood flow which can lead to serious cardiovascular disorders such as heart attack.

Red meat is capable of disrupting the hormone balance in your body by elevating the levels of estrogen. This can lead to endometriosis, a disorder of the uterine muscles, which can be very painful and pose serious reproductive complications in the long term. Such estrogen dominance can even lead to cancer associated with hormone imbalance such as uterine or breast cancer.

The problem is greater when you consume factory-farmed meat or stored meat available at supermarkets which contains preservatives and harmful chemicals that can dysregulate your entire physiological system. Such kind of meat also contains endocrine disruptor substances such as phthalates and other organic pollutants which can totally shift the working of your hormonal system and microbiome in the wrong direction.

This is why you need to avoid consuming red meat on the whole and specifically factory-farmed and market-bought stored meat. But you don't need to worry, there are many healthy alternatives to red meat such as eggs and fatty fish which are enriched with Omega-3 fatty acids that can shift your hormonal balance towards improvement.

Processed food

Although canned and processed foods may be an easy and 'ready-to-go' option for you but do you know how harmful these instant meals can be for your biological system? You may love these convenient food options but your hormones surely hate them. It is natural for hormone levels of your body to fluctuate during different phases of your cycle but unusual hormonal imbalances are not natural. They are triggered by harmful chemical substances which are very likely to be present in processed foods.

One such ingredient found in these on-the-go foods is added sugar. This does not account for natural sugars present in frozen fruits and vegetables. We are pointing to the extrinsic sugars like fructose which are added to processed foods for the purpose of flavoring and preservation. These artificial sugars can disrupt the level of insulin hormone in your body, which can ultimately lead to complications, and worsening of symptoms of PCOS.

You may know very well that these processed foods mostly come in plastic packaging which is itself very harmful due to its composition. Apart from being destructive for the environment, plastics can be extremely harmful for your health as well. Plastics contain Bisphenol A which interferes with your body's hormone cycle causing destruction in production, storage, transportation and normal functioning of hormones. However, there is no need to be sad about how much processed food you have consumed in the past. What's done is done. But now you can take control. Start by reducing your intake of highly processed foods like snacks, cake bars, crisps, instant noodles, and carbonated drinks. Make simple swaps in your daily routine like trading a supper chocolate snack bar with some fresh fruits or juices and there you go with processed foods far away from your life!

Caffeine

Do you love coffee? I do too. But is it good for you? I don't think so. You daily cup of morning freshness may not be as refreshing for your hormones. Coffee is notorious for its main active component that is caffeine. Caffeine can interfere with the normal levels of various hormones in your body. These include estrogen, progesterone, testosterone, cortisol, serotonin and dopamine.

Latest scientific research has shown that caffeine has the ability to impede normal functioning of estrogen in your body. However, this notion is different for women belonging to different races. For Asian and African women, caffeine causes an increase in levels of estrogen while for White women, estrogen levels may drop in case of excessive caffeine intake. In one way or the other, caffeine does disrupt normal levels of estrogen and can lead to increased risk of hormonal complications associated with estrogen imbalance.

As estrogen and progesterone levels are interrelated, disturbance in estrogen levels can impact progesterone balance as well. These disproportions can worsen symptoms of hormonal imbalance like heavy or absent periods, painful menstruation, hirsutism, acne and sudden weight gain.

Caffeine also interferes with the balance of cortisol in your body. Cortisol being a stress hormone manages your mood and stress levels. Taking caffeine boosts cortisol levels which are already disturbed in case of hormonal imbalance and can further make your body go into a level of high alertness leading to further hormonal problems.

Yes, we know that suddenly dropping coffee from your everyday routine is not possible and we don't suggest that either. But you have to start somewhere. Start by replacing your morning cup with a less caffeinated option like some lemon or green tea. You have to make this difficult dietary change if you want to stay healthy because sometimes the change we resist the most is the change we need the most.

Soy products

Considered to be a unique food that presents many positive health effects, soy can be harmful for your hormone balance if taken in excessive amounts. This nutrient-rich source of protein has caused conflicting views when it comes to its ability to disrupt hormonal balance. Although many researchers have construed soy to be a good dietary addition with amazing nutritional benefits but many have shunned it for its potential for causing disturbance in estrogen levels of your body.

Soy contains phytoestrogen that can function as estrogen in the body leading to very high levels of this hormones. Such estrogen dominance can lead to very harmful complications like breast and colorectal cancer as well as imbalance of estrogen/progesterone ratios which can ultimately worsen symptoms of hormonal imbalance like irregular menstruation, painful periods, anxiety and mood swings.

The disturbance in your menstrual and ovulation cycle caused by excessive intake of soy can hamper your potential of getting pregnant as well.

Soy being a very common part of American cuisine is very hard to avoid but it is essential that you consume soy products like tofu, tempeh, soy sauce, and soy milk in moderate amounts which cannot interfere with your hormone balance or further worsen an existing hormonal imbalance problem.

Dairy products

Have you ever wondered that all the cheese and milk you consume excessively might be the cause of your hormonal problems? This may not be the same for every woman. Some female bodies have amazing ability to digest and metabolize milk and milk products but for some these dairy items may be harmful when consumed unreasonably.

Milk and other dairy products contain hormones like estrogen, progesterone and insulin-like growth factor 1. If you consume dairy products in large amounts then the levels of these hormones in your body may become very high leading to hormonal imbalance and problems like irregular menstruation, infertility, extreme menstrual cramps, mood swings, irritability, acne, hirsutism, weight changes, hot flashes during menopause and endometriosis.

The ability of dairy products to disrupt hormonal balance can lead to severe complications like cancer of the breast, uterus or ovaries. Thus, consuming dairy products can further worsen any kind of hormonal imbalance already present in your body.

We are not saying that you need to totally cut off dairy from your life. No, that's not the case. Dairy has its beneficial impacts as well when consumed in moderate amounts. We are just emphasizing on the notion that the excess of everything is bad. So, the best suggestion here would be to start reducing your intake of dairy products by opting for some fibrous alternatives like chia and flax seeds and taking other healthier sources of calcium and proteins like coconut, nuts, and oats.

Certain vegetables

Cruciferous vegetables belong to the family Brassicaceae and include cauliflower, kale, broccoli, brussels sprouts, turnip greens and cabbage. People suffering from hormonal imbalance need to keep a check on their consumption. The same goes for vegetables belonging to the Nightshade family such as brinjal, peppers, potatoes and tomatoes. Just like dairy and soy products, these vegetables are good for your hormones if consumed in moderate amounts but excessive intake can lead to harmful effects on your hormone regulation system.

Both these types of vegetables have the ability to mess with your thyroid functioning where they reduce the amount of iodine in your body leading to hypothyroidism or severe complications of the thyroid hormones T3 and T4. This could lead to problems like enlarged thyroid gland (goiter), heart problems, infertility, mental health problems, cancer and birth defects in newborn babies of pregnant females.

Women already suffering from hypothyroidism and related hormonal issues really need to have a second thought on their consumption of these vegetables. Despite their amazing nutritional value, they may be problematic when used in excessive amounts.

6. CYCLE SYNCING

We women always feel like we are a slave to our hormones. This ever-changing system of chemical messengers has us at its beck and call. You are happy at one point and suddenly your mood shifts to a sad phase of crying and sulking. All because of this unstable and dynamic cycle of hormones and menstruation. Scientific research has shown that you may feel different in different phases of your menstrual cycle. This is due to the hormonal fluctuations that occur all throughout your cycle making you feel content in the middle of the month whereas sad, anxious and depressed before your period. These hormonal shifts control your moods, emotions and your overall body responses. It is high time you take over control and stop being a victim to this ferocious cycle of change. This is where the importance of cycle syncing arises.

WHY IS CYCLE SYNCING IMPORTANT?

The term 'cycle syncing' was first introduced by Alisa Vitti who described this phenomenon in her book Woman Code based on her nutritional and hormonal expertise. Cycle Syncing is a way to hack your menstrual cycle. It is when you adapt or change your daily life processes like your diet, physical activity, sexual routine, and even social or work engagements to coincide with different phases of your menstrual cycle. In this way, you are capable of supporting your body as per its requirements throughout your monthly hormonal shifts.

Cycle syncing is a way of harnessing your hormonal energy and cyclical powers for further enhancing your well-being, creativity and health satisfaction. This new trend of biohacking not only helps manage your moods and cravings as per hormonal shifts but switching up your eating ad exercising habits in different phases of your cycle can also help you lose weight.

However, there are many things you need to consider before starting cycle syncing. Irrespective of whether you want to cycle sync to manage mood swings, for alleviating fatigue due to PMS, loosing weight or if you want to become pregnant, it is essential that you consult with your health care provider. It is essential to know your body's current state before making any changes in your physical or dietary routine and to know whether cycle syncing is an efficient course of action for you or not. A sound decision in consultation with your physician can greatly help you in converting your cycle of emotional fluctuations to a cycle of self-care, contentment and well-being.

WHO CAN BENEFIT FROM CYCLE SYNCING?

Every woman can gather fruit from the beneficial tree of cycle syncing in one way or the other. However, this phenomenon may be especially helpful in the following cases:

- If you are trying to get pregnant

- If you are experiencing a decreased sex drive
- If you have an irregular menstrual cycle
- If you have Poly Cystic Ovary Syndrome (PCOS)
- If you are struggling with symptoms of PMS like mood swings, abdominal cramps, acne, weight gain, or bloating
- If you have very painful and heavy periods every month
- If you are overweight
- If you feel extraordinarily lazy or fatigues throughout the month
- If you want to balance your hormones after giving birth
- If you want to balance your hormones after getting off birth control pills or IUD
- If you want to get rid of hormonal acne

In all of the above situations, cycle syncing can be very helpful in managing hormonal fluctuations and making your body adapt to these changes without causing a disturbed state of mind. Scientists claim that cycle syncing can benefit you in many different ways such as:

- Increases your energy levels
- Lessens mood swings and episodes of anxiety and depression
- Alleviates menstrual cramps
- Regularizes your period cycle
- Enhances your chances of conceiving
- Aids in losing weight
- Makes your workout routine more effective
- Supports in management of PCOS
- Makes you feel healthy and active

All these benefits of cycle syncing and yet you are making your body suffer from all those emotional rollercoasters every month. This wonderous biological maneuver can benefit every woman who menstruates and experiences mood swings and unwanted health issues during different phases of her monthly cycle.

FRAMEWORK FOR CYCLE SYNCING

To begin with cycle syncing you first need to know the phases of your menstrual cycle and how this system works. The menstrual cycle of hormonal shifts spans over a period of four weeks and includes four different phases i.e., follicular phase, ovulatory phase, luteal phase and menstrual phase.

The follicular phase is the period prior to release of egg in the uterus. Ovulatory phase includes the process of egg release and luteal phase includes the hormonal changes occurring after the egg is released. Menstrual phase is the name given to the time your period occurs. Here is a breakdown of how long every phase of your cycle is and what hormonal changes occur during each phase:

Phase	Approximate duration	Hormonal changes	Emotional state
Menstrual Phase (part of follicular phase)	1-5	Follicle stimulating hormone (FSH) and estradiol are on the rise and progesterone and estrogen levels are low.	Your energy levels are low and you may feel fatigued
Follicular Phase	6-14	Estrogen and progesterone levels begin to rise	You may feel energetic, inspired and happy

Ovulatory Phase	15-17	Estrogen levels are highest. Progesterone, testosterone, estradiol increases and luteinizing hormone (LH) is released	Your sex drive and libido increase and you might feel the need to look more attractive
Luteal Phase	18-28	Estrogen and progesterone levels are on the rise. The body prepares lining of uterus for implantation of embryo and if egg is not fertilized the cycle starts again.	You feel intense mood swings, anxiety, and food cravings

However, the above-mentioned hormonal and emotional changes are not fixed. Every woman is different and every body responds differently to hormonal fluctuations. The days for which each phase lasts are also not fixed. This is a guideline for you to track the phases of your cycle and understand the framework of cycle syncing.

HOW TO START CYCLE-SYNCING?

The first step to start cycle syncing begins with getting to know your own body and how your body changes in every phase of your cycle. Get in touch with your body, know your eating routines and see how your natural rhythms fluctuate throughout the month. Understand the changes in your energy levels during each phase of your cycle and take note of your cravings and eating habits. So, observation is the first step towards cycle syncing.

Next, you need to track the length of your cycle. You need to know how long your cycle lasts so that you can split and identify it into phases and function accordingly. You can track you cycle by noting the first day of your period on the calendar and counting days until your next period comes. Track these days for several months until you get an idea about the approximate length of your cycle. You can also track your cycle by using various apps such as MyFlo, Clue and Spot On.

Once you have tracked your cycle, then you can begin to change your eating habits for every phase of your cycle accordingly. Start with small changes and replacements until you develop a healthy routine. Similarly, you can modify your exercise routine to fit with the requirements of every phase of your cycle. In this way, you can protect your body from straining itself and reasonable physical activity that is consistent with your cycle supports you in losing weight and staying fit. Then you can also focus on managing your work engagements during every phase of your cycle. Don't impose excessive work on yourself and strain your mind in the second half of your cycle where the hormonal changes already have your energy levels low. Try to manage you social and official time in ways you feel more content and comfortable.

SEED CYCLING FOR HORMONE IMBALANCE

Seed cycling is a new and effective way of syncing your hormonal cycle in a natural way. It is a very simple technique that requires little effort yet has a big impact on your hormonal regulation system. It is a way of benefiting from the healing powers of natural seeds and incorporating them in your daily routine to maintain hormone balance, prevent irregular periods, boost fertility and alleviate problematic PMS symptoms like anxiety, painful cramps, heavy flow, and mood swings.

The practice of consuming specific types of seeds during two halves of your menstrual cycle is called seed cycling. This promotes the hormonal balance of progesterone and estrogen. When followed consistently this practice can help maintain a regular menstrual cycle, stimulate absent periods and enhance your chance of conceiving. Every woman can benefit from seed cycling irrespective of age or weight. Even post-menopausal women can utilize this biological way of balancing their hormones and prevent complications related to hormone imbalance in old age.

If you are just coming off birth control or suffering from symptoms of post-birth control syndrome like irregular periods or acne, then seed cycling can greatly help you in reviving your hormonal balance.

How to use seeds for hormonal balance?

The process of seed cycle is very simple and easy to understand and follow. All you have to do is use pumpkin and flax seeds during the first 14 days of your cycle and take sunflower and sesame seeds in the last 14 days of your cycle. Here's a breakdown of the amount and type of seeds you need to take to maintain hormone balance through seed cycling:

- Day 1-14 (Menstrual and follicular phase): Take 1-2 tablespoons of flax seeds and 1-2 tablespoons of pumpkin seeds every day.
- Day 15-28 (Ovulatory and luteal phase): Take 1-2 tablespoons of sunflower seeds and 1-2 tablespoons of sesame seeds every day.

If you don't have a cycle that lasts 14 days then there is no need to worry. All you have to do is follow this process for 14 days and it will automatically sync your cycle to the optimal natural biological rhythms.

If you have an irregular menstrual cycle and your period is missing for some months than you have to follow the seed cycling phases according to the phases of the moon in the following manner:

- Day 1-14 (New moon to full moon): Take 1-2 tablespoons of flax seeds and 1-2 tablespoons of pumpkin seeds every day.
- Day 15-28 (Full moon to new moon): Take 1-2 tablespoons of sunflower seeds and 1-2 tablespoons of sesame seeds every day.

This may seem odd or superstitious but it actually works because of the ability of the moon to impact center of gravity. It actually impacts your hormonal cycle because the moon cycle is also 28 days and a balanced hormonal cycle also lasts for 28 days.

How seed cycling impacts every phase of your cycle?

The nutritional properties and components of pumpkin, flax, sesame and sunflower seeds play a vital role in managing hormone balance through seed cycling. Let's discuss how seed cycling can benefit every phase of your cycle individually:

- Menstrual and follicular phase: flax seeds help maintain the estrogen levels in follicular phase and prevent estrogen dominance by binding of their components (lignans) with excess estrogen. Pumpkin seeds are packed with zinc which help support progesterone balance.
- Ovulatory and luteal phase: sesame seeds and sunflower seeds have the ability to enhance production of progesterone as they are enriched with zinc, selenium and vitamin E which detoxify your reproductive system and maintain hormonal balance.

How to sync your sexual routine with your cycle?

A woman's sexuality is a topic as taboo as menstruation. Normalizing conversations about feminine sexuality is as important as the need to spread awareness about menstruation. Despite the social, political and technological achievements women have made over the past decades, they still feel ashamed and hesitate while talking about their sexual and menstrual problems.

Just like hormonal fluctuations impact your moods, dietary routine and physical activity, they also impact your libido and sex drive. Changes in hormonal levels during different phases of your cycle impact how you behave sexually and can increase or decrease your desire for sex. Let's discuss some tips for managing your sexual routine during different phases of your menstrual cycle:

Menstrual phase: Most women experience cramps and fatigue during this phase. Although scientific research shows that orgasms and sexual pleasure may help relieve cramps but it always depends on you and your desire. Its better to rest during this time and eat healthy so that you can gear up for the next phase of your cycle.

Follicular phase: During this phase, hormonal fluctuations cause your sex drive to lessen and you don't feel tempted or attracted at all. We suggest you to resort to small foreplay (massaging or touching) rather than penetration because keeping it slow helps keep you at ease.

Ovulatory phase: The levels of estrogen and progesterone are highest during this time and so is your sex drive. it is the ideal time to try for a baby if you want to become pregnant. Keep things fiery and exciting at this time so that you can benefit fully from the surge of hormones that occurs in your body.

Luteal Phase: Your sex drive is low during this phase as compared to ovulatory phase. You may want to try some loving techniques and slightly more stimulation to achieve full satisfaction, climax and an ultimate state of pleasure.

CYCLE SYNCING AND THE INFRADIAN RHYTHM

You might not have heard about this before but your menstrual cycle is governed by a specialized biological rhythm called the infradian rhythm. The term 'infra' means beyond and 'dian' means a day. So, infradian rhythm is a bodily cycle or rhythmic pattern that extends beyond a day. It refers to a bodily process that extends beyond a period of one day or

24 hours. Your 28-day hormonal cycle is actually an infradian rhythm which is a very important part of female hormone health and every woman experiences this rhythm monthly through her cycle. The key to heal a hormonal imbalance is knowing what your body needs in terms of diet, nutrition, physical activity and emotional insight.

A clear understanding of what the infradian rhythm is and how it affects your body is very important before starting cycle syncing. There are two biological time managers, one is the 24-hour circadian rhythm and second is the infradian rhythm. The circadian rhythm is experienced by both men and women. However, the infradian rhythm is only a part of female physiology and only women or people with female physiology experience it. However, only women who are in their reproductive years experience the infradian rhythm.

The infradian rhythm greatly regulates the four phases of the reproductive cycle of females but it is not the only system of your body affected by infradian rhythm. This biological timekeeper has a global affect in your body and it affects six systems of a female body. These include:

- Central nervous system
- Metabolic system
- Immune system
- Reproductive system
- Microbiome
- Stress response system

The infradian rhythm affects the female physiology in a cyclical way which is why it is important that your body's needs should also be addressed in a cyclical way. Therefore, females should coincide their daily life activities like eating, moving, sex, social activities with their infradian rhythm so that they can live an optimal and healthy life.

7. CYCLE SYNCING FOR MENSTRUAL PHASE

HORMONAL CHANGES DURING MENSTRUAL PHASE

As you know that your monthly menstrual cycle is divided into four phases i.e., the menstrual phase, follicular phase, ovulatory phase and luteal phase. Menstrual phase is the first phase of your cycle. We are sure you are very aware of this phase as it is the annoying aunty flow, also known as your period, who pays a haunting visit every month. You might be aware of the basics of what does your period mean but it is important to have an insight on where does this phase stand in your cycle, what is happening with your hormones in the background and how it affects your body.

When does the menstrual phase occur?

The menstrual phase occurs at the very start of your monthly cycle and includes the initial 1-5 days of your period.

What happening?

Menstruation is the name given to your body's way of eliminating the thick uterine lining, also known as endometrium, through your vagina. This process occurs when the egg released by ovaries and implanted into the uterus is not fertilized and the thickened uterine lining is no more required to protect the fertilized egg and it begins to shed. The vaginal discharge that occurs during your period consists of broken tissues of the uterine lining, mucus, and blood. In this phase, hormonal levels of estrogen and progesterone begin to drop. Estrogen levels drop to the lowest point just before your period.

What physical symptoms do you experience?

You are very likely to experience some uncomfortable symptoms during your period which include:

- Breast tenderness
- Abdominal cramps
- Lower back pain
- Mood swings
- Irritability
- Fatigue
- Bloating
- Dizziness

What happens to your brain?

The hormonal changes occurring during menstrual stimulate the functioning of your brain. In this case, the left part of your brain which is responsible for analytical functions and the right part of your brain which is responsible for your feelings coordinate very strongly. This means that your brain is active and it is the ideal time to express your feelings or make a decision for which your have been thinking for some time. This is the best time where you can reflect your thoughts and feelings or journal if you like to.

How can you manage your period?

The vaginal discharge that occurs during your period can be very messy and problematic if not managed properly. You need to use sanitary pads or tampons to absorb it and ensure good hygiene to avoid infections and unwanted hygienic problems like vaginal itching and rashes.

What should be your goal?

During this phase your body is going through a process of detoxification and blood loss. Your goal should be to boost your iron levels by consuming iron rich foods and reducing inflammation. You should give your body time to heal. Take some rest and allow your muscles and nerves to relax.

What should you avoid?

Avoid overstraining your body with intense exercises and too much physical activity. Limit intake of high-sugar and processed foods. Avoid cold and frozen dietary items like ice creams, slushes and cold drinks.

SOME FACTS YOU MIGHT NOT KNOW ABOUT YOUR MONTHLY PERIOD

Do you think that your period can surprise you with a visit only when you least expect it? Nope, we don't think so. On an average every woman experience about 450 periods during her lifetime. We think that's quite enough time to know all what there is to know about. But we are sure there are some interesting hidden facts about your period which you are still not aware of. Let us uncover them for you:

Getting pregnant during your period is possible

Its high time that the age-old myth that your period can protect you from conceiving should be squashed. There are some reasons why you could get pregnant. The female physiology is very complex and unpredictable. Sometimes women bleed when they are in the ovulatory phase of their cycle. They can mistakenly perceive the bleeding to be their period and having sex during this time can in fact, increase the chances of getting pregnant because it is the most fertile time of your reproductive system.

Another reason can be the fact that sometimes a new egg may be released before your period ends and the sperm is capable of surviving in a female body for 2-3 days. Therefore, having sex during your period can lead to pregnancy. So, ladies if you don't want to become pregnant then don't take the cover of your periods, rather be sure to take birth control pills or use protection while having sex irrespective of the time of the month.

The period you get while taking birth control pills is actually not a true period

The bleeding that occurs when you take birth control pills is actually not your period rather it is something called 'withdrawal bleeding'. This kind of bleeding is a bit different from your period. As you might have read in the previous section of the chapter, normally, your period occurs when the egg in your uterus is not fertilized and the thickened uterine lining begins to shed. Birth control pills prevent your body from releasing an egg but they do not stop the uterine lining from building up. So, the bleeding that occurs during the last week of taking birth control pills is not due to absence of a fertilized egg but due to the absence of hormones that occurs when you take these pills which makes this bleeding different from your period.

The span of your menstrual cycle changes with age

Your hormonal system is an ever-changing cycle of twists and turns. It is very likely that the span of your menstrual cycle may change over time and as your age increases. During early stages of puberty, you cycle is usually longer and the time span between two periods is longer. The menstrual cycle of a teenage girl lasts for about 21 to 45 days. However, as age advances, the cycle becomes shorter and its average length ranges from 21 to 35 days.

As a woman nears menopause, the hormonal changes in her body become very unpredictable and her period may get heavier or lighter and the time span between two period may become shorter or longer. These changes may begin even 10 years before you have your menopause. But these slight hormonal changes in the body are a part of your normal physiology.

There are many new and innovative choices other than the regular pads and tampons

The age-old traditions of using sanitary pads and tampons are now outdated. Innovation has brought forward some new and easier ways of managing your period. These include menstrual cups, period panties, sea sponges and many more.

A menstrual cup is a very soft and flexible cup that can fit inside your vagina and gather all the period blood which you can discard and reuse the cup after cleaning it with boiling water.

A period panty is a superabsorbent underwear which you can wear with comfort. It has a layer that absorbs blood. the panties offer a lot of comfort are available in many sizes and absorbency levels and can even be washed and reused.

A period sea sponge is exactly what its name suggest. It is used just like a menstrual cup and is placed inside your vagina to absorb the period blood. they are available in many sizes depending upon the intensity of your flow and you can easily wash and reuse them.

OPTIMAL FOODS FOR MENSTRUAL PHASE

Do you crave some ooey-gooey, chocolaty snacks and some salty, spicy crisps during your magic lady time? These cravings might seem very comforting while watching your favorite Netflix show during aunty Flo week but actually consuming these unhealthy foods during your period can worsen your symptoms and cause many problems. Let us tell you some foods you need to redefine those 'good stuff' cravings if you want to cycle sync your menstrual phase and keep those hormones in balance.

During your period your body loses a lot of blood and it requires iron to make new and fresh red blood cells. A moderate amount of lean red meat can help you add that needed iron in your body. If you are a vegetarian then there's no need to worry about. Vegetables like spinach, zucchini, eggplant, broccoli and chard also contain iron and so do some lentils and beans.

You body also needs antioxidants during this time to fight off toxins and free radicals which can cause problems like cancer and diabetes. You can consume antioxidants from sources like raspberries, blueberries and cherries.

Fibers are a good thing to eat during menstrual phase to keep your body safe from estrogen dominance and to prevent inflammation. Sweet potatoes, cauli flower, brussels sprouts, apples, grapefruits and whole weight granola are amazing sources of fiber.

Omega-3 fatty acids and B vitamins are also essential nutrients you need to fight period cramps and for muscle relaxation. Fatty fish like salmon are very good sources of these nutrients and protein as well.

For beverages, a hot cup of lemon or green tea can really help freshen your mind, relax your body and alleviate those problematic period cramps which can be very irritating and painful. Some chamomile tea can also help relieve anxiety, relaxes your nerves and also helps you sleep peacefully so that you wake up with a fresh start to a new day.

PHASE-SPECIFIC RECIPES

1. Buckwheat granola

If you love granola and are fed up of the commercial expensive granolas which contain gluten and high-sugar content then you are going to love this easy buckwheat granola. This portable breakfast option is very rich in nutrients, gluten-free and perfect to keep your sugar levels in check during your period.

Course: Breakfast
Cuisine: American
Preparation time: 10 minutes
Cooking time: 20 minutes

Ingredients:

- Buckwheat groats – 2 cups
- Sunflower seeds – ¼ cup
- Pumpkin seeds – ¼ cup
- Shredded coconut – ¼ cup
- Cranberries – ¼ cup
- Ripe mashed banana – 1
- Coconut oil – 2 tablespoons
- Maple syrup or honey – 2 tablespoons
- Nutmeg – ½ teaspoon
- Cinnamon – ½ teaspoon
- Salt – a pinch

Instructions:

Add all your ingredients in a large bowl and mix them thoroughly to cover everything. Line baking tray with butter paper and spread all the mixture over the tray very evenly. Heat this in a preheated oven at 300 °F 20-25 minutes. Make sure to stir your mixture occasionally and keep checking to protect it from burning. Then remove your mixture from the pain and allow it to cool at room temperature for about 15 minutes. Break the granola into chunks and store it in a resealable bag or air tight container. You can use it up to 2 weeks.

2. **Warm eggplant curry with chickpeas**

Eggplants and chickpeas have the ability to enhance your digestion by boosting the production of bile and stomach acid which not only reduces bloating during periods but also helps treat abdominal cramps. Here is a warm and cozy eggplant quinoa recipe with chickpeas than can boost your digestion and make your gut healthy.

Course: Entree
Cuisine: Ayurvedic
Preparation time: 10 minutes
Cooking time: 40 minutes

Ingredients:

For the quinoa:

- Quinoa (plain or sprouted) – 1 cup
- Bone broth (any kind of meat) – 2 cups
- Cardamom – 3 pods
- Star anise – 1-2 pieces

For the curry:

- Large eggplants (peeled and diced) – 2 large
- Chickpeas (rinsed and drained) – 1 large can
- Large onion (diced) – 1
- Garlic (minced) – 4 cloves
- Ginger (chopped) – 1 tablespoon
- Fresh cilantro (chopped) – 1 bunch

- Tomato paste – ¼ cup
- Coconut oil – 2 tablespoons
- Coconut milk – 2 cups
- Coriander powder – 3 teaspoons
- Cumin powder – 3 teaspoons
- Turmeric – 2 teaspoons
- Sea salt – 2 teaspoons
- Cardamom – 1 teaspoon
- Cinnamon – 1 teaspoon
- Fennel – ½ teaspoon
- Black pepper – to taste

Instructions:

Start making the quinoa by boiling the bone broth with quinoa in a pot and then add cardamom and star anise to the pot. Cover it and let it simmer for 15 minutes until all moisture is absorbed. Cover and steam it for another 10 minutes. Then fluff it with a fork and remove the star anise and pods before serving.

Take another pan and melt the coconut oil in it. Add in the diced onion and cook on medium heat until translucent. Add garlic and ginger to it and cook for a minute then add all the rest of the spices and let it cook and fry for another 2-3 minutes on medium heat until fragrant. Add the tomato paste and stir the mixture for another 2-3 minutes. Add the eggplants and cook for additional 2-3 minutes. Toss the chickpeas into the pain and add coconut milk. Bring the mixture to a boil and then let it simmer for 20-30 minutes until the eggplant softens. Add a cup of chopped cilantro and keep the rest for garnishing. Dish out and serve it with the quinoa.

3. Spicy meatball curry with coconut and lamb

Who doesn't love a good dish of spaghetti and meatballs? I'm sure you do. But the regular combo of spaghetti and meatballs is not a healthy dietary option if you are trying to balance your hormone levels. Here is a recipe of an amazing meatball curry with coconut and lamb which has a hint of spice and all the good nutrient properties of healthy protein and vitamins which help balance your hormones during menstrual phase.

Course: Main course
Cuisine: American
Preparation time: 10 minutes
Cooking time: 50 minutes

Ingredients:

For meatballs:

- Lamb (minced) – 1 pound
- Green onion (diced) – ¼ cup
- Cilantro (chopped) ¬– ¼ cup
- Ginger (grated) – 1 tablespoon
- Garlic – 1 teaspoon
- Curry powder – 1 tablespoon
- Sea salt – ½ teaspoon
- Pepper (ground) – to taste
- Sesame oil – 1 teaspoon
- Coconut oil ¬– 2 tablespoons

For coconut sauce

- Coconut milk (full-fat) – 14 ounces
- Cashew butter – 1/4 cup
- Soy sauce – 1/4 cup
- Curry powder – 2 tablespoons
- Maple syrup or honey – 2 teaspoons
- Garlic (chopped) – 1 teaspoon
- Ginger (chopped) – 1 teaspoon

- Siracha sauce –– to taste (based on the spice level you like)
- Sesame oil – 1 teaspoon

For noodles:

- Low carb veggie noodles/ brown rice noodles – 1 medium-sized packet
- Cilantro (chopped) –– for garnishing

Instructions:

Make the noodles by coking them in boiling water for 10-12 minutes. Then strain them and set aside. While the noodles are cooking, start working on the meatballs. Mix together all ingredients of meatballs in a large bowl and make the mixture into medium-sized meatballs by hand. Make the sauce by mixing all ingredients in blender until the consistency becomes creamy. Set the sauce aside. Now add 2 tablespoons of coconut oil in a stovetop pan of medium heat. Place the meatballs on the pan and cook them until brown on each side. Now cover the meatballs in the sauce and cook it in a preheated oven at 350 °F for 15 minutes. Serve this meatball curry over your noodles and top it with fresh chopped cilantro. Enjoy!

4. Cinnamon and almond smoothie

Being on a cycle-syncing diet for hormone balance doesn't mean you have to skip on sweet and cool refreshing drinks. This cinnamon and almond smoothie is the perfect kick you need to boost your energy levels and get also those nutrients in.

Course: Drink
Cuisine: American
Preparation time: 5 minutes
Cooking time: 5 minutes

Ingredients:

- Non-dairy milk – 1 cup
- Almonds ¬(raw) – 10
- Dates (pitted) – 4
- Coconut oil – 1 teaspoon
- Cinnamon (ground) – 1 teaspoon
- Ice cubes – 2

Instructions:

Add all the ingredients into a blender and blend for about one minute. Transfer to a glass and serve right away.

5. Salty peanut butter balls

Every woman has the right to fulfill her sweet craving during periods. But eating the unhealthy high-sugar chocolates is not the best thing to do. Here is a very sweet and healthy alternative which is actually nutritious and also fulfills all your cravings for something sweet and delicious.

Course: Dessert or snack
Cuisine: American
Preparation time: 5 minutes
Cooking time: 30 minutes

Ingredients:

- Low-fat peanut butter – 2 cups
- Dark chocolate – 1 and a ½ cup
- Maple syrup or honey – ½ cup
- Coconut flour – ¼ cup
- Collagen powder – 4 tablespoons
- Coconut oil (melted) – 1 tablespoon
- Sea salt – ½ tea spoon

Instructions:

Add the peanut butter and maple syrup to a large bowl and mix them thoroughly by vigorous stirring. Now add the coconut flour and collagen powder to the bowl and mix everything. Stir in the sea salt. Now roll the mixture with your hands into small bite-size balls and set them aside. Now melt the chocolate in coconut oil over low heat while continuously stirring. Use a fork to dip and coat each ball in the chocolate. Set the balls on a trap with parchment paper. Drip the remaining chocolate over the balls. Top off with some sea salt and place the balls in the freezer for 10-15 minutes to make them firm. Serve and enjoy!

6. Peanut and sweet potato stew

Sweet potatoes and peanuts contain all the necessary vitamins and fibers you need to boost your health while you are on your period. The healthy fat content of this dish supports your body's energy needs and keeps your gut healthy.

Course: Main course
Cuisine: African
Preparation time: 10 minutes
Cooking time: 20 minutes

Ingredients:

- Coconut oil – 2 tablespoons
- Onion (chopped) – 1
- Ginger (minced) – 1 tablespoon
- Garlic (chopped) – 4 cloves
- Sea salt – 1 teaspoon
- Cumin – 1 teaspoon
- Siracha – 1 teaspoon
- Black pepper – ¼ teaspoon
- Low-fat peanut butter – ¾ cup
- Tomato paste – ½ cup
- Bone broth – 3 cups
- Coconut milk – 1 cup
- Red bell pepper (chopped) – 1
- Spinach (chopped) – 2 cups
- Sweet potatoes (chopped) – 2
- Fresh cilantro – for garnishing

Instructions:

Sauté the onions on a stove top pan in coconut oil on medium heat for 5-10 minutes until translucent. Add the salt, black pepper, ginger, cumin and garlic to the pan and mix and cook for 2-3 minutes until fragrant. Now add the bone broth, peanut butter, tomato paste, bell pepper, sweet potatoes, siracha and coconut milk. Stir the mixture until everything is combined thoroughly. Cover the pot and turn the heat to high until the stew begins to boil. Them simmer it for 15-20 minutes on low heat until the sweet potatoes become soft. Now turn off the heat and add in the greens. Serve it with your favorite choice of grains (brown rice or quinoa). Enjoy!

PHASE-SPECIFIC EXERCISES

Your hormone balance is very specifically linked to the physical activity and exercise you do on a daily basis. This is because exercising impacts metabolism which in turn regulates the functioning of your hormonal cycle. Therefore, changes in your exercise routine can disturb your hormonal balance. In order to cycle sync for hormone balance it is essential to plan your workouts and physical activity according to the requirements of your body in every phase of your cycle. This not only makes your workouts more productive but also helps prevent exercise from disrupting your hormone balance.

Menstrual phase is the most slow and tiring phase of your cycle. During this time, you might want to just chill and rest. Let your body have some time to heal and focus on just light walks or slow and meditative yoga. Let's have a look at some exercises you can do during this phase of your cycle.

Slow, meditative walks

A light walk in the park while listening to your favorite playlist can greatly help relieve your anxiety and relax your muscles while alleviating the cramps you feel during periods. Some light stretching and hiking can also help your hormones during this phase.

Yin yoga

Yin is a kind of slow-paced yoga. It is very meditative and known for its ability to relieve tension, reduce stress, alleviate anxiety, relax your muscles and make your mood instantly happy and induce a sense of well-being. It also helps improve your bone health and softens stiff joints. It involves some slow log-held poses involving mostly the extremities and lower part of your body like hips, legs, pelvis, feet and thighs. The poses are usually held for five minutes and everything is done slowly and peacefully which can also help improve your body's flexibility and blood circulation.

Kundalini yoga

Unlike in yoga, kundalini yoga is a rather intense and spiritual form of yoga which involves intense poses, breathing, meditation and loud changing or singing. Kundalini refers to the energy which is trapped or coiled in your spine. Doing kundalini yoga helps activate this energy which can benefit you in many ways. It helps reduce stress and enhances your level of pain tolerance. It improves your mood and cognitive behavior, manages optimal blood sugar levels and enhances body flexibility.

8. CYCLE SYNCING FOR FOLLICULAR PHASE

HORMONAL CHANGES

The next phase in your menstrual cycle is the follicular phase. It is often referred to as the "spring" phase of your cycle where the ovaries are working to produce an egg. The follicular phase actually overlaps with the menstrual phase. The menstrual phase of your cycle is considered to be a part of the follicular phase and some scientists consider the follicular phase to be of 14 days starting from the first day of your period until the start of ovulation. If you want to know how your hormones change during follicular phase, how your body is affected physically and emotionally during this phase and how you can optimize your eating habits to support hormonal balance then read on.

When does the follicular phase occur?
The follicular phase usually begins from the next day your periods end and lasts up to the 14th day of your cycle until ovulation occurs.

What's happening?
The follicular phase begins with the release of follicle stimulation

hormone (FSH) from the pituitary gland. This hormone is responsible for triggering the ovaries to produce and mature about 5-20 follicles each of which contains an immature egg. Most of the time only the healthiest egg will go on to become completely mature. In very rare cases, two eggs can become mature which if fertilized can lead to twin babies. The rest of the follicles containing immature eggs are reabsorbed by the body. Now the maturation of the follicle containing the egg causes a rise in levels of estrogen, which prompt the uterine lining to become thick for implantation of fertilized egg. This occurs in order to create a nutrient-rich and safe environment inside the uterus for the embryo to grow. At this time, the ovaries are ready to release the egg, which occurs in the next phase of the menstrual cycle. The length of follicular phase can vary in different women but the average length is about 6-7 days.

What physical symptoms do you experience?

During the follicular phase, your body's metabolism is generally slower and the levels of cortisol are lower in resting phase. The surge in hormones that occurs after your period ends causes an increase in your energy levels. You are very likely to feel energized, happy and in your form. You skin feels glowing, your body feels light and good and your sex drive also increases during this phase. Suddenly, you feel very confident and assertive and the urge to do something adventurous is highest during this time.

What happens to your brain?

The increase in estrogen levels that occurs during follicular phase cause your brain to become more active. Your cognitive functions improve and you begin to think more clearly. New ideas of exploring things begin to pop in your mind. Symbolically, we can surely say that this is the phase of creativity, confidence and new beginnings.

What should be your goal?

As you feel very pumped and energized during this phase then it is the best time to start working on your life goals. If you want to lose weight then get moving. It is the best time of the month to train your body and build your muscles. Your goal should be to utilize this energy as much as possible to benefit your physical and emotional health as much as possible.

What should you avoid?

Smoking and alcohol abuse are the worst things you can do to your body during any phase of the menstrual cycle. The maturation of follicles and eggs in your ovaries can be negatively affected by the influence of alcohol and toxic nicotinic components of cigarette. This is especially important if you are trying to conceive. Smoking and alcohol abuse can hamper your fertility and endanger the safety of eggs in your ovaries. Therefore, you must avoid consuming alcohol and cigarette smoke during this phase.

OPTIMAL FOODS FOR FOLLICULAR PHASE

During the follicular phase your body needs essential nutrients like omega-3 fatty acids, phytoestrogens, fibers, proteins, minerals like magnesium and foods which can strengthen your reproductive system and help support the maturation process of eggs that occurs during this phase.

Healthy fats like omega-3 fatty acids are capable of balancing the level of FSH hormone in your body which is the most prominent hormone of follicular phase. Imbalance of this hormone can disrupt the follicular phase and in turn the following phases as well which is why consuming these healthy fats during follicular phase is very important. Foods rich in omega-3 fatty acids include fatty fish like salmon, avocado, egg yolk, seeds like pumpkin and flax seeds, nuts like almonds and peanuts and oils like olive and avocado.

Phytoestrogens are plant-based estrogen-balancing substances that can help prevent estrogen dominance in your body which is associated with symptoms like irregular periods, mood swings, anxiety, bloating and other hormonal issues. Consuming phytoestrogens can help balance estrogen levels during follicular phase. Foods containing phytoestrogens include some vegetables like collard green, garlic, radish and watercress. Other sources of phytoestrogens include tofu, tempeh, flax seeds and sesame seeds.

The hormonal changes occurring during follicular phase disrupt the levels of different minerals in your body, which are required for many physiological functions. One of these minerals is magnesium. Magnesium also helps metabolize excess estrogen in the body thus preventing estrogen dominance. It is important to consume more magnesium during follicular phase to prevent tis deficiency and complications associated with it. Foods rich in magnesium include vegetable greens, nuts (hazel nuts, almonds), whole grains (wheat flour, brown rice, quinoa) and beans (kidney, garbanzo).

Prior to ovulation, your body undergoes a lot of oxidative stress as well. In order to combat this, you should incorporate foods rich in vitamin C, which is the best antioxidant fights stress-causing free radicals. Such foods include citrus fruits like lemon, oranges, and grapefruit, berries, zucchini, bell pepper, broccoli, cabbage and bok choy.

Other than all these specific nutrients, it is essential to generally include moderate amounts of carbs, fiber and proteins in order to meet all the nutrient requirements of your body. Carbohydrates rich in fibers are a good dietary component when consumed reasonably. High fiber carbs can be found in fruits like grapes, kiwi and oranges, vegetables like squash, sweet potatoes, potatoes, parsnips and carrots, legumes like beans and lentils, and whole grains like wheat flour and quinoa. Protein foods to include high-quality protein in your diet include fresh and organic chicken breast, tofu, and legumes.

Intake of probiotics in your diet can also help neutralize your microbiome and regulate hormone balance during follicular phase. Organic sources of probiotics include sauerkraut, kimchi and pickles.

PHASE-SPECIFIC RECIPES

1. Zucchini oatmeal

Zucchini is originally a fruit but it is mostly served in cooked form. It contains all the essential nutrients like vitamin C and antioxidants, which your body needs during follicular phase. And when paired with oatmeal, it is the best combo for incorporating fibers and nutrients in your breakfast.

Course: Breakfast
Cuisine: American
Cooking time: 10 minutes
Preparation time: 5 minutes

Ingredients:

- Oats (rolled) – ¼ cup
- Zucchini (grated) – ¼ cup
- Almond milk – ½ cup
- Eggs (only whites) – 2
- Collagen powder – 1 tablespoon
- Almond butter – 1 tablespoon
- Coconut oil – 1 tablespoon
- Cinnamon (ground) – 1 teaspoon
- Vanilla extract – 1 teaspoon
- Salt – to taste

Instructions:

Take a medium-sized sauce pan and place it on the stove and keep the heat medium. Add all ingredients into the pan and cook everything for about 10 minutes while stirring continuously until everything is thoroughly combined. You can add milk or water to make the consistency up to your desired level. Serve and enjoy!

2. Balancing chipotle and cauliflower tacos

These hormone-balancing chipotle and cauliflower tacos are considered to be the best vehicles for transporting nutrients and components which boost your hormone regulation system without depriving your taste buds of some amazing flavors. The ingredients of this recipe contain all the detoxifying nutrients that help balance hormone levels during follicular phase.

Course: Entrée
Cuisine: Mexican
Cooking time: 10 minutes
Preparation time: 30 minutes

Ingredients:

For the tacos:

- Cauliflower (coarsely chopped) – 1
- Avocado oil – 4 tablespoons
- Garlic (chopped) – 4-6 cloves
- Chipotle sauce – 2 teaspoons
- Maple syrup or honey – 1 tablespoon
- Cilantro (chopped) – 1 cup
- Lime juice – 1 tablespoon
- Black pepper (crushed) – to taste
- Salt – to taste

For chipotle aioli:

- Low fat mayonnaise – ½ cup
- Sour cream – ½ cup
- Chipotle sauce – 1/4 cup
- Garlic (chopped) – 2 cloves
- Sea salt – 1 teaspoon

For serving and topping:

- Almond flour-based tortillas
- Chopped tomatoes, cucumber, radish, and red cabbage
- Chopped guacamole

Instructions:

Spread the coarsely chopped cauliflower florets on to a baking sheet lined with parchment paper. Toss over 2 tablespoons of avocado oil and add the chopped garlic, salt and black pepper evenly over the florets. Roast it in a preheated oven at 350 °F for 30-35 minutes while flipping the florets halfway through the time. While the florets are roasting, take a separate bowl and add the remaining ingredients of the tacos i.e., chipotle sauce, avocado oil, cilantro, maple syrup or honey and lime juice. Mix everything together thoroughly and set the bowl aside.

Take another bowl and add all the ingredients of the chipotle aioli and mix them well together. Set the bowl aside. Once the cauliflower is well roasted mix it with the remaining ingredients of the cauliflower. Serve this mixture in tortillas and top of with the chipotle aioli and other toppings of your choice. Serve and enjoy!

3. Winter green pizza

Do you love pizza? We are sure the answer is yes. Who doesn't love pizza? But regular pizza is a very unhealthy food choice which is not good for your hormones. We have brought for you a very healthy and nutritious recipe for pizza which is sure to fulfill all your pizza cravings without harming your hormones from all the excess pizza calories.

Course: Main course
Cuisine: Italian
Cooking time: 1 hour
Preparation time: 10 minutes

Ingredients:

For pizza crust:

- Tapioca flour – 2 cups
- Coconut flour – 1/3 cup
- Olive oil – ¼ cup
- Egg – 1
- Water – 1-2 cup

For pesto pizza sauce:

- Garlic (chopped) – 1 tablespoon
- Pumpkin seeds (sprouted) – 1/4 cup
- Arugula – ¼ cup
- Lemon (juiced) -1
- Extra virgin olive oil – ½ cup
- Sea salt – to taste
- Crushed black pepper – to taste

For toppings:

- Butternut squash (chopped) – 2 cups
- Onion (finely sliced – ½ cup
- Garlic (chopped) – 1 teaspoon

- Fresh spinach – 1-2 cups
- Almond-milk ricotta cheese – as per your liking
- Pomegranate seeds – ¼ cup
- Olive oil – 4 tablespoons
- Sea salt, black pepper and red chili flakes – to taste

Instructions:

Place the butternut squash and onions on a baking tray. Drizzle over olive oil and add garlic, salt and pepper. Roast it in a preheated oven at 425 °F for about 30 minutes and flip it after half time. Line two large pizza pans with parchment paper. Make the pizza crust by mixing all the ingredients in a large bowl and slowly add water add knead until the consistency becomes doughy. Divide the dough in two sections and place each on parchment paper and sprinkle some coconut flour on top. Place another sheet of parchment paper on top. Use a rolling pin to roll out the dough very thin. Place the doughs on the two lined pizza pans. Bake them at 450°F for 15 minutes.

While the dough is baking, make the pesto sauce by blending all ingredients together thoroughly at a high speed. Remove the crust from the oven and turn the heat down to 400 °F. Now top your pizza with the pesto sauce, olive oil, roasted squash, spinach, onions and cheese. Let the pizza bake at 400 °F for 30 minutes until golden brown. Now add the pomegranate seeds, arugula, salt, pepper and lemon juice over the pizza. Serve and enjoy.

4. Superfood-loaded fries

Loaded fries are a latest and very popular fast food. We are sure love them two. But the regular and traditional loaded fries are packed with very unhealthy carbs and high-calorie fats which are not at all good for your hormones. Here we present you a recipe for loaded fries which is enriched with healthy ingredients that contain all the necessary nutrients and minerals you need during follicular phase.

Course: Entree or snack
Cuisine: American
Cooking time: 10 minutes
Preparation time: 5 minutes

Ingredients:

For top-load:

- Avocados (ripe) – 4
- Kale (chopped) – 1-2 cups
- Onion (finely chopped) – ½ cup
- Cilantro –1/4 cup
- Jalapeno (finely sliced)– 1
- Yellow bell pepper (chopped)– ½ cup
- Garlic (minced) – 4 cloves
- Lemon (juiced) – 1
- Salt – to taste
- Black pepper – to taste

For fries:

- Jicama (peeled and cut into sticks for fries) – 1
- Lemon juice – 2 tablespoons
- Sea salt – to taste
- Chili powder – to taste

Instructions:

Place the kale in a basket and steam it in a pot of boiling water for about 2-3 minutes until it turns bright green. Remove it from the basket and allow it to dry by placing it on a kitchen towel and patting dry. Allow it cool and finely chop it. Mash the avocados in a bowl and add the rest of the ingredients of the top load. Mix everything together thoroughly. Add the chopped kale and mix again.

Take the jicama fries and drizzle the lime juice, salt and chili powder on top. Serve the fries in a bowl and add the top-load. Enjoy!

5. Fudgy fertility-boosting smoothie

If you are trying to eat healthy but can't cut down on the heavy smoothies you love then there is no need to worry about. We have a recipe for you that has all the added nutrients like healthy fats, minerals, proteins, fiber, leafy greens all in a non-fatty liquid base. Surprising, right? The nutritional benefits of this smoothie don't just end here. The nutrient-rich components of this smoothie have immense fertility-boosting properties and it can greatly aid you in your journey towards a healthy pregnancy.

Course: Drink
Cuisine: American
Preparation time: 10 minutes

Ingredients:

- Unsweetened, low-fat nut milk – 1 cup
- Chocolate-flavored protein powder – 2 tablespoons
- Flaxseeds (ground) –1 tablespoon
- Cacao powder – 1 tablespoon
- Cacao nibs – 1 tablespoon
- Cinnamon (ground) – 1 teaspoon
- Sea salt – ½ teaspoon
- Dates (pitted) – 1-2
- Small avocado (peeled) – ½
- Nut butter (any kind of your choice) – 1 tablespoon
- Any leafy green of your choice (kale, spinach or Swiss chard) – 1 handful
- Cauliflower – ½ cup
- Banana – ½

Instructions:

Blend all ingredients together at high speed until everything becomes trough combined and creamy. Add some ice cubes if you want to and enjoy!

6. Oat crumble bars

If you love a nice and healthy dessert then these oat crumble bars are for you. They are packed with high-fiber oats and home-made strawberry filling that can provide all the essential nutrients and fibers you require to optimize you diet for follicular phase.

Course: Dessert or breakfast
Cuisine: America
Cooking time: 30 minutes
Preparation time: 10 minutes

Ingredients:

For the crust:

- Almond flour – 1 cup
- Oat flour (gluten-free) – 1 cup
- Rolled oats (gluten-free) – ½ cup
- Coconut (grated) – ¼ cup
- Coconut or olive oil – 3 tablespoons
- Coconut sugar or honey – 3 tablespoons
- Flax paste – 1 tablespoon powdered flax seeds mixed in 3 tablespoons of water

For filling:

- 2/3 cups home-made strawberry jam

For crumble topping

- Rolled oats – ½ cup
- Honey – 1 tablespoon
- Coconut oil – 1 tablespoon
- Leftover oat crust

Instructions:

Make the flax paste by mixing together the flax seed powder in 3 tablespoons of hot water. Set it aside. Melt the honey and coconut oil by putting them in a small bowl and microwaving for 30 seconds. Add all the ingredients of the crust in a large bowl and mix them evenly. Take 3/4th portion of the oat crust and place it in a baking pan lined with parchment paper. Press the crust in the pan evenly with your hands. Pour the strawberry jam over the crust and use a spatula to spread it evenly in to the pan. Mix up the crumble top ingredients in a bowl and crumble them over the jam. Place the pan in a preheated oven at 350 °F for 30 minutes or until the crumble becomes golden brown. Remove it from the oven and let it cool to room temperature. Cut it into bars or any shape you like. Serve and enjoy!

PHASE-SPECIFIC EXERCISES

The energy level of your body is quite high in this phase and you should take the most advantage out of it, it is the best time to push yourself for some intense strength training, HIIT and cardio. Here are some of the exercises you can do to boost your hormone balance during follicular phase:

High-intensity Interval training (HIIT)

If you are fitness freak then you must be very well aware of what HIIT is. It includes very fast and energy-requiring exercises that are very fun to do. The high energy levels of your body during follicular phase make it a perfect time to do some HIIT. It helps normalize your body's hormone levels and boosts natural energy stores and ability to burn calories.

Strength training

The follicular phase of your cycle is one of the best times to boost your body's strength ability and push yourself to do some strength training. This means that what you need to do in follicular phase is to replace the knee push-ups in your exercise routine with toe push-ups. Use heavier weights while lifting. And if you are new to strength training then there is no need to worry about. You can begin with some bodyweight exercises and try to build up your workout confidence so you can avail the energy of this phase to the highest potential.

Cardio

Cardio is a kind of exercise which boosts your heart rate and pushes your body to use energy and burn calories. The follicular phase is the best time to do some cardio exercises and boost your body's hormonal balance. Some of the best cardio exercises that you can do include jumping jacks, skipping, squats, sit-ups, running, boxing, hiking, biking and swimming.

Flow-based yoga

Flow-based yoga is a very peaceful and energizing form of yoga. It involves a lot of physical movements like dancing, standing and various poses along with heavy breathing, meditation, balancing and inversions. It improves your body's flexibility, ability to manage stress and utilize stored energy to burn calories.

9. CYCLE SYNCING FOR OVULATORY PHASE

HORMONAL CHANGES DURING OVULATORY PHASE

After the follicular phase has ended your body begins to enter the 'summer' phase of its cycle. This is the ovulation phase and as the name suggests it involves the release of the egg, which was matured in the follicular phase. This is the prime time for baby-making as your reproductive system is at the peak of its fertility potential. There are many hormonal changes that occur during this phase and impact your physical and emotional health. Let's have a look into the details of this phase:

When does the ovulatory phase occur?

Ovulatory phase begins the next day follicular phase ends. It usually starts on the 15th day of your cycle and lasts till the 17th day. However, this may vary in different women between 12th-17th day due to the different lengths of their cycle. The ovulatory phase typically lasts for about 2-3 days only.

What's happening?

The ovulatory phase begins just when the rise in levels of estrogen stimulate the hypothalamus to release the gonadotropin-releasing hormone (GnRH). This hormone then triggers the pituitary gland to start releasing luteinizing hormone (LH). Within two days, the surge in LH levels causes the mature follicle containing the egg to burst and release the egg. This egg has a very short lifespan. If not fertilized, it will disintegrate within 12-24 hours.

The cervix begins to move upwards to allow the egg to be fertilized by sperm. This is the best time to have sex if you are trying to conceive. The sperm is required to move upwards through the cervix which becomes soft during this phase and travel to the egg. Only the fittest sperm can survive this and fertilize the egg. The egg travels from the follicle towards the uterus by the movement of small hair-like projections. If it fertilized by a sperm during this time then it gets implanted in the uterus otherwise, the egg dies. At this point your body experiences the highest levels of estrogen and testosterone which also influence your emotional and physical health.

What physical symptoms do you experience?

During the ovulatory phase your body goes through a lot of hormonal changes and the intense process of the fertilization of egg. It is likely that you may feel a slight rise in your basal body temperature. Your vaginal discharge can become white and thick like the consistency of an egg. You may feel slightly moody and lethargic in some cases. Some women also experience constipation and a slight rise in their body weight which is probably just the water weight.

What happens to your brain?

The shift of hormones that occurs in ovulatory phase triggers the social and verbal parts of your brain. You might feel more communicative and wanting to socialize with people around you. This also incites more confidence in you so if you have been wanting to talk about something important with someone for some time but couldn't, then this is the time my friend.

What should be your goal?

The ovulatory phase is the most fertile time of your cycle. If you have been wanting to conceive then there is no other best time. Get that sexy energy going because the fertility window is not going to stay open for long. It is highly likely for you to feel more attractive during this time so go and make a move. However, if you don't want to get pregnant than be extra cautious while having sex during this phase.

What should you avoid?

Try to avoid foods rich in carbs like pasta, chips, cakes and pastries. You should not consume sodas or fizzy drinks that are highly carbonated. Reduce your intake of caffeine and try to avoid alcohol intake and smoking. Cut down on sugar, red meat and processed foods and if you a couch potato then start moving but do not engage in extremely heavy physical activities or lifting.

OPTIMAL FOODS FOR OVULATORY PHASE

As your estrogen levels are quite high during ovulation, it is important to eat foods which can detoxify your body from excess estrogen and prevent problems associated with estrogen dominance. Such foods include cruciferous vegetables like broccoli, brussels sprouts, cauliflower, turnip, kale and cabbage. Other detoxifying foods include guava, strawberries, coconut and raspberries which aid the liver in detoxification of excess hormones by improving the quantity of glutathione.

Being the most fertile period of your cycle, you might want to include fertility-boosting nutrients in your diet if you want to get pregnant. These nutrients include vitamin B6, omega-3 fatty acids, folic acid, and choline. Foods rich in these fertility-enhancing nutrients include kidney beans, whole grains like quinoa and buckwheat, mushrooms, sesame seeds, sunflower seeds, green leafy vegetables, organic red meat, and fatty fish like salmon and sardines.

You should also incorporate fiber-rich foods and probiotics in your diet to help support your gut health and keep the microbiome functioning properly. These foods include organic yoghurt, whole grains like wheat flour, quinoa and brown rice, non-starchy vegetables, legumes, beans like kidney and garbanzo and nuts like almond, peanut, and hazelnuts.

Your body also essentially requires proteins during this phase. Try to gain protein from fish sources or plant sources and avoid animal-based sources of proteins. This is because animal protein includes some toxic chemicals, which interfere with hormonal balance and can hamper your chances of conceiving. Opt for plant-based protein sources like tofu, beans (kidney, garbanzo), nuts (almonds, hazelnuts, cashews, peanuts), seeds like chia, basil, sunflower and sesame seeds. Eggs can also serve as a good source of protein during this phase. Fish that are low in levels of mercury are also good sources of protein for ovulatory phase. Examples include salmons, tuna and sardines. But they should be consumed in moderate amounts. Some fish varieties that you should essentially avoid during this phase include sword fish, king mackerel and tilefish because they are rich in mercury and can damage your hormone balance and endanger your fertility potential.

PHASE-SPECIFIC RECIPES

1. Grain-free porridge

If you want to add some healthy porridge to our diet but don't like grains then this recipe is surely for you. It is based on seeds and nuts and is a very low-carb diet that helps in weight loss and managing hormone balance during ovulatory phase.

Course: Breakfast
Cuisine: American
Preparation time: 5 minutes
Cooking time: 10 minutes

Ingredients:

- Almond milk – 1 cup
- Hemp hearts – 1 tablespoon
- Almond butter – 1 tablespoon
- Chia seeds – 1 tablespoon
- Cashew nuts – ¼ cup
- Cinnamon (Ground) – 1 teaspoon
- Vanilla extract – 1 teaspoon
- Berries and fruits of your choice for topping

Instructions:

Put all ingredients except the toppings in a blender and blend them at high speed. Pour the blend in a stove top pan and warm it. Top off with fruity toppings of your choice. Serve warm and enjoy!

2. Grilled salmon and avocado salad

Summers are arriving and you surely need some easy and refreshing recipes to beat the heat. Featuring some of summer's best vegetables in combination with the healthiest protein source i.e., salmon, topped off with an amazing sweet and salty miso sauce, is an amazing meal packet with all the nutrient-rich properties required by your body during the ovulatory phase.

Course: Entrée
Cuisine: Asian-fusion
Preparation time: 10 minutes
Cooking time: 10 minutes

Ingredients:

For salmon:

- Fresh salmon fillet – 1
- Butter (from grass-fed poultry) – 2 tablespoons
- A pinch of garlic powder, sea salt, black pepper, chili powder and paprika

For the salad:

- Spinach – 4 cups
- Avocado (peeled and diced) – 1
- Cucumber (chopped) – 1
- Asparagus (ends removed) – 1 bunch
- Avocado oil – 1 tablespoon
- Sea salt – to taste
- Black pepper – to taste
- Cilantro (chopped) – 1 cup

For miso dressing:

- Olive oil – ½ cup
- Lemon juice – ¼ cup
- Vinegar (organic) – ¼ cup
- White miso paste – ¼ cup
- Honey and maple syrup – ¼ cup
- Garlic (chopped) – 1 teaspoon
- Sea salt – 1 teaspoon
- Black pepper (crushed) – to taste

Instructions:

Take the asparagus, toss it in the avocado oil, and sprinkle some salt and pepper. Grill it over medium heat on a pre-heated grill on both sides for about 5 minutes. Marinate the salmon fillets with butter and other seasoning and place them on the grill. Cook them for about 6 minutes on each side or until your desired level of rawness. As the salmon and asparagus are on the grill, take the ingredients of the miso dressing and put them in a blender. Blend at high speed until a smooth puree is formed. Set it aside. Now take a large bowl and add the remaining ingredients of the salad. Add the grilled asparagus. Top it with the miso dressing. Add the grilled salmon on top. Serve and enjoy!

3. Herbalicious fertility-boosting smoothie

Organic and natural herbs along with green leafy vegetables are a woman's best friend if she wants to become pregnant and boost her health for a better preconception phase and healthy pregnancy. This smoothie is filled with all the fertility-boosting foods you can think of and is sure to convert your reproductive system into a baby-making machine.

Course: Drink
Cuisine: American
Preparation time: 10 minutes

Ingredients:

For nut milk:

- Brazil nuts (raw) – 1 cup
- Filtered drinking water – 2 cups
- Dates (finely chopped) – 2-4
- Vanilla extract – 1 teaspoon
- Sea salt – a pinch

For the smoothie:

- Nut milk – 1 or 1 ½ cups
- Spinach (frozen) – 1 handful
- Kale (frozen) – 1 handful
- Vanilla-flavored protein powder – 1 medium scoop
- Almond butter – 1 tablespoon
- Chia seeds – 1 tablespoon
- Dates (chopped) – 1-2
- Spirulina powder – 1 teaspoon
- Avocado (chopped) – ¼
- Banana (frozen) – ½

Instructions:

For the nut milk, soak all the ingredients together in a bowl for 8 hours or overnight. Then add them to a blend and blend at high speed until everything is thoroughly combined. Now strain the mixture and set aside. Take all the ingredients of the smoothie in a blender. At the nut milk and blend together at high speed until the mixture become thick, smooth, creamy and thoroughly combined. If you find the smoothie very thick you can thin the consistency by adding more nut milk. Top it off with your favorite healthy dressings. Serve cool and enjoy!

4. Keto-friendly bacon chowder

Looking for a low-fat healthy meal which is easy to make and not time-consuming? Your have reached the right page of the book. This bacon chowder is filled with all the goodness of healthy fats and proteins. it is not only nutritious but very flavorful as well and can fulfill all your savory cravings. It is also very beneficial if you are on a keto diet.

Course: Main course
Cuisine: American
Preparation time: 10 minutes
Cooking time: 40 minutes

Ingredients:

- Cauliflower (coarsely chopped) – 1 large unit
- Avocado oil – 2 tablespoons
- Organic bacon – 8 strips of half inch each
- Yellow onion (chopped) – 1
- Carrot (diced) – 1
- Celery (diced) – 1 cup
- Organic bone broth – 2-3 cups
- Low-fat coconut milk – 1 cup
- Parmesan cheese (optional) – ½ cup
- Organic ghee – 2 tablespoons
- Garlic (chopped) – 4 cloves
- Thyme leaves (fresh) – 1 tablespoon
- Bay leaf – 1
- Sea salt – 2 teaspoons
- Chili flakes – to taste
- Black pepper (crushed) – to taste

Instructions:

Place the florets of the chopped cauli flower on a baking pan lined with parchment pepper. Drizzle them with avocado oil and add half of the garlic, salt and black pepper. Roast hem for about 30 minutes until they are golden burn and flip after half of the time. chop the bacon strips and cook them in a saucepan over medium heat until it turns crispy. Transfer the bacon to a plate and set it aside. To the same pan add the ghee and melt it. Add the diced onion to the pan and cook it on medium heat util it turns translucent. Now add garlic, salt, pepper, chili flakes and thyme. Mix everything together and cook for one minute. Now add the diced celery and carrot and cook it for several minutes until it softens. Now gradually star adding the bone broth and keep stirring until you get the perfect consistency. Bring the mixture to a boil and then let it simmer on low heat. Now add the roasted cauliflower florets to this and mix together everything. Let is simmer for 15 minutes on low heat. Remove it from the heat and add the coconut milk and optional parmesan cheese. Now add the bacon to the mixture and stir it. Top off with some cilantro and serve warm. Enjoy!

5. Strawberries and cream parfait for seed cycling

As discussed in the previous chapters of this book, seed cycling is an amazing way of managing hormone balance naturally. This delicious creamy parfait is field with the goodness of strawberries and all the amazing seeds which can help boost your reproductive functioning during ovulatory phase.

Course: Dessert
Cuisine: American
Preparation time: 10 minutes
Cooking time: 30 minutes

Ingredients:

For the seed granola:

- Organic cashews – 1 cup
- Organic almonds or walnuts – 1 cup
- Coconut flakes (unsweetened) – 1 cup
- Organic sesame seeds – 1 cup
- Organic sunflower seeds – 1 cup
- Cinnamon (ground) – 1 teaspoon
- Sea salt – to taste
- Coconut oil – 2 tablespoons
- Maple syrup or honey – 1/3 cup
- Vanilla extract – 1 teaspoon

For the parfait:

- Coconut yoghurt (unsweetened) – 2 cups
- Organic strawberries (sliced) – 1 cup
- Any toppings of your choice (pistachios, whipped cream, berries, coconut flakes)

Instructions:

Take a baking sheet and line it with parchment paper. Take all the nuts of the granola in a chopper and pulse chop them until a chunky and crumbly texture is obtained. Add the coconut flakes and pulse again to mix everything. Transfer the pulsed mixture to a bowl and add the remaining dry ingredients i.e., sesame and sunflower seeds and sea salt. Take all the wet ingredients in a separate bowl and mix them well together by using a whisk. Pour the wet mixture into the dry ingredients and mix everything together. Spread this mixture evenly over the lined baking sheet and bake it in a preheated oven at 325 °F. When halfway through, stir the mixture over without breaking the clusters. Bake until it turns golden brown from both sides. Remove from the oven let the granola cool at room temperature. Start assembling your parfait in glass jars. Start with a layer of granola the bottom the toss in some coconut yoghurt followed by sliced strawberries. Repeat the layers and at the end add the toppings of your choice. Serve and enjoy!

6. Green pulpy muffins

Do you know that all the nutritional benefits of leafy greens are in its pulp? Yup, that's right. But we know that most of the time you just discard the purple and strain the green juice. That is not nutritionally beneficial at all. We have brought you a recipe for some yummy vegan muffins that preserve the pulp of greens and all their nutrient goodness.

Course: Dessert/breakfast
Cuisine: American
Preparation time: 15 minutes
Cooking time: 30 minutes

Ingredients:

- Oat flour (gluten-free) – 1 and ½ cup
- Pulp of vegetable greens (kale, cauliflower, broccoli, brussels sprouts) – 1 cup
- Honey or maple syrup – ¾ cup
- Extra virgin olive oil – 1/ cup
- Almond butter – 4 tablespoons
- Desiccated coconut – 4 tablespoons
- Organic apple cider vinegar – 1 teaspoon
- Baking powder – ½ teaspoon
- Baking soda – ½ teaspoon
- Sea salt – ¼ teaspoon
- Vanilla extract – 1 teaspoon

Instructions:

Preheat your oven at 375 °F. Add all the dry ingredients in a large bowl and mix them thoroughly. Take all the wet ingredients in a separate bowl and whisk them together. Now gradually add the wet ingredients to the dry ingredients and combine them well with the help of a spatula. Take a muffin tray and line it with muffin liners. Portion out the batter into the tray. Pat the tray on your counter to even out the batter and remove air pockets. Bake the batter for about 35 minutes. Remove from the oven and allow to cool at room temperature. Serve and enjoy!

PHASE-SPECIFIC EXERCISES

Just like the follicular phase, the ovulatory phase is also a period of high energy levels. During this time, you should push your body for intense workouts like HIIT and high-intensity cardio so that you can make the most out of this energy-rich, fertile phase. here are some workouts which can help in your hormone balance and fulfill your body's needs during the ovulatory phase:

High intensity interval workouts

As discussed above for the follicular phase, you can try the same HIIT workout you do for the follicular phase in this phase as well. If you want to push yourself harder than go for circuit training or other kinds of strength training which build up your muscles and boost your body's metabolism and calorie-burning capacity. Other high intensity workouts which can help you during this phase include kickboxing, swimming, running, fast-paced jogging, rowing, climbing and hiking.

Spin class

A spin class is the name given to group exercises where the focus is placed on full-body workouts, strength training, and resistance-based intervals. It involves indoor cycling which greatly helps in improving your heart function, strength, endurance and has a positive impact on your hormonal health as well. It is amazing for weight loss too.

10. CYCLE SYNCING FOR LUTEAL PHASE

HORMONAL CHANGES DURING LUTEAL PHASE

Also known as the "fall" season of your cycle, luteal phase is the last phase of your menstrual cycle. This phase is where your body decides if its going into a new cycle or into pregnancy. This totally depends on if the egg is fertilized or not. Your energy levels begin to fall during this phase and there is a surge in the level of sex hormone progesterone. Your body begins to prepare itself for a new menstrual cycle and there come the most dreaded symptoms of a premenstrual syndrome (PMS).

When does the ovulatory phase occur?
The luteal phase begins on the 18th day of your cycle and lasts for about 10 days until the 28th day. It starts right after ovulation and lasts until the start of your next period.

What's happening?
The follicle from which the egg is released stays on the surface of the

ovary for some time. The follicle then begins to cluster into a mass called the corpus luteum. This mass begins to release progesterone and small amount of estrogen as well. These hormones cause the uterine lining to become thick and prepare the uterus for the implantation of the fertilized egg. If the egg become fertilized then a new hormone called the human chorionic gonadotropin (hCG) is released in your body which further thickens the uterine lining and also helps maintain the corpus luteum keeping it intact. Pregnancy tests usually detect the presence of this hormone to confirm pregnancy.

However, if the egg is not fertilized then the corpus luteum begins to shrink and dissolve and it reabsorbed into the body. As result, progesterone and estrogen levels begin to drop as result of which the uterine lining begins to shed away. This causes the onset of PMS symptoms and makes your energy levels drop. The shedding of uterine lining causes the onset of menstruation and hence the cycle repeats.

What physical symptoms do you experience?

The estrogen and progesterone levels reach their peaks during the luteal phase and then begin to drop when the egg is not fertilized. This drop in hormone levels causes your energy levels to drop as well due to changes in the level of serotonin hormone. Serotonin is the hormone that manages your mood so low level of serotonin is the culprit behind the unwanted PMS symptoms. You may feel fatigued and lethargic. Symptoms of PMS emerge as result which include mood swings, abdominal cramps, irritability and intense cravings for fatty and sweet foods.

What happens to your brain?

The low energy levels during this phase also affects your brain. You are likely to feel low and irritable. Socializing feels like a huge task and you might want to stay at home alone and rest. The PMS symptoms also mess with your brain causing mood swings and fatigue along with sleep disturbances.

What should be your goal?

This is a phase of intense mood swings and low energy levels. Your goal should be to give your body some time to rest and replenish your energy levels by taking nutrients and stabilizing your hormones with a good diet. You can fulfil the intense food cravings by taking your comfort food on and off. Let your body and mind rest so that you can prepare for menstruation which is coming as the next cycle starts.

What should you avoid?

Try to avoid foods that can further burden your body during this slow phase. Such foods include alcohol, caffeine and highly processed sugars. Avoid burdening your body and overstraining yourself with intense workouts.

OPTIMAL FOODS FOR LUTEAL PHASE

The strengthening of uterine lining is the most important physical change occurring in your body during luteal phase. As this process id driven by the release of progesterone, it is important to eat foods that stimulate the production of progesterone in your body. Nutrients like vitamin C and B6, zinc and magnesium greatly help in promoting the levels of progesterone. Nuts (almonds, peanuts and cashews), beans and seeds (sesame and sunflower) are the best sources of zinc and magnesium. Citrus fruits (grapefruit, oranges and lemon) and green leafy vegetables are the best sources of vitamin C. Vitamin B6 can be consumed from foods like salmon, walnuts and dates.

It is important to maintain a good nutrient-rich diet during the luteal phase in order to keep your sugar levels in balance which are often tipped off by decreasing hormone levels and PMS. This is what causes PMS cravings as well. Try to eat foods that are healthy and rich in good fibers, proteins and carbohydrates.

Water retention is a common problem during this phase which can cause problems like bloating. Try to drink as much water as possible to keep yourself hydrated. Increase the consumption of hydrating fruits like watermelons.

We know that you feel intense sweet-cravings during the luteal phase because of a drop in your "feel-good" hormone, serotonin. Do not reach for unhealthy sweet snacks to fulfil your cravings. Opt for healthy alternatives like protein bars and a small amount of dark chocolate that can fulfil your cravings without the unhealthy sugar dump.

Try to incorporate those foods in your diet that can boost your serotonin levels as it make your mood better. Examples of such foods include quinoa and buckwheat.

PHASE-SPECIFIC RECIPES

1. Millet porridge

If you're looking for a nutrient rich breakfast to substitute the tasteless oatmeal you don't like then this millet porridge is the best option for you. It is the perfect combination of healthy grains from millets and fresh fruits that can provide most of the nutrients you require during the luteal phase.

Course: Breakfast
Cuisine: American
Preparation time: 5 minutes
Cooking time: 5 minutes

Ingredients:

- Almond milk ¬– ½ cup
- Millet seeds (ground) – 2 large tablespoons
- Organic cinnamon (ground) – 1 teaspoon
- Vanilla extract – ½ teaspoon
- Your favorite fruits for topping

Instructions:

Take all ingredients except the toppings in a stovetop pan and mix them thoroughly. Cook for five minutes until the mixture is thoroughly combined and warmed. Serve in a bowl and top off with your favorite sliced fruits. Enjoy!

2. Sweet potato pesto bowl for healthy gut

A healthy gut is essential for maintaining hormone balance. This sweet potato pesto bowl is no only insanely flavorful but contains all the gut-friendly nutrients like omega-3 fatty acids, vitamin B6, healthy fats, whole grain fibers and good proteins which help maintain your gut health and keep your hormones in balance.

Course: Entrée/ main course
Cuisine: American
Preparation time: 10 minutes
Cooking time: 35 minutes

Ingredients:

For the pesto:

- Basil – 2 cups
- Arugula – ¼ cup
- Pistachios (shells removed) – ¼ cup
- Lemon juice – 1 tablespoon
- Sea salt – 1 teaspoon
- Garlic (minced) – 2 cloves
- Black pepper (ground) – to taste
- Extra virgin olive oil – ½ cup

For the bowl:

- Quinoa (sprouted and cooked) – 1 cup
- Organic eggs – 2-4
- Sweet potatoes (sliced like fries) – 1-2
- Avocado (chopped) – 1
- Sea salt – to taste
- Black pepper – to taste
- Chili flakes – to taste
- Avocado oil – 2 tablespoons
- Garlic (minced) – 2 cloves
- Dill and chives – for topping

Instructions:

Take a large baking sheet and line it with parchment paper. Place the sliced sweet potatoes on the baking sheet and drizzle the avocado oil over them. Sprinkle some salt, pepper and chili flakes on top. Bake them in a preheated oven at 425 °F for about 30 minutes and flip them after half the time. Now, start working on the pesto. Take all the pesto ingredients in a food processor and mix them on high speed until everything is thoroughly combined. Set it aside. Cook your eggs as you desire. You can either fry, boil, poach or scramble them as per your liking. After everything is cooked, start assembling your bowl. Add the quinoa to the bowl first followed by the sweet potatoes, eggs and avocado. Now add the pesto on top. Top it off with some fresh chives and dill. Serve warm and enjoy!

3. Herb-loaded sweet potato nachos

Nachos are everybody's favorite snack and if you are in the PMS phase then you must be craving them a lot. But the regular nachos you eat are full of bad carbs and not a healthy option for your hormones. Here we present to you a healthy recipe for nacho cravings that is nutritious and delicious at the same time.

Course: Snack/entrée

Cuisine: Mexican
Preparation time: 5 minutes
Cooking time: 35 minutes

Ingredients:

For nachos:

- Sweet potatoes (thinly sliced rounds) – 2 medium-sized units
- Avocado oil – 2-4 tablespoons
- Chili powder – 2 teaspoons
- Paprika – 1 teaspoon
- Garlic powder – 1 teaspoon
- Sea salt – ½ teaspoon

For toppings:

- Dairy-free healthy cheese
- Black beans (cooked)
- Rotisserie chicken (organic)
- Guacamole
- Lettuce, tomatoes, jalapenos and radish (thinly sliced)
- Cilantro (chopped)

Instructions:

Line a baking tray with parchment paper. Coat the sliced sweet potatoes with avocado oil and rest of the spices. Place them with even spacing on the lined baking tray and bake in a preheated oven at 425 °F for about 30 minutes while flipping halfway through. After the halfway flip sprinkle the cheese on each slice of the sweet potatoes and let it melt as the slices are baking.

Once the nachos are done, remove them from the oven and place them in a dish. Top off with the black beans and chicken and broil in the oven for about 1-2 minutes. Remove from the oven and add the remaining toppings of your choice. Serve warm and enjoy!

4. Maple-coated stuffed squash boats

This recipe of delish squash boats is sure to trick all those people who hate healthy eating. It is packed with amazing flavors of squash, vegetables, a little bacon and a drizzle of maple syrup to make it the perfect amount of sweet and savory.

Course: Entrée / main course
Cuisine: American
Preparation time: 5 minutes
Cooking time: 30 minutes

Ingredients:

- Squash (medium-sized) – 2
- Sweet onion (chopped) – ½
- Organic and unprocessed bacon – 4-6 slices
- Kale leaves (chopped) – 1 bunch
- Pecans (raw) – ¼ cup
- Pomegranate seeds – ¼ cup
- Avocado oil – 4 tablespoons
- Garlic (minced) – 4 cloves
- Sea salt – to taste
- Cumin – 1 teaspoon
- Cloves – 1/ teaspoon
- Black pepper (crushed) – to taste
- Maple syrup – for drizzling

Instructions:

Cut each squash lengthwise into two sections. Scoop out the seeds. Line a baking tray with parchment paper. Place the squash cut side down on the lined tray and drizzle with avocado oil, salt, and pepper. Bake in a preheated oven at 425 °F for 30 minutes or until the squash becomes tender.

Take a large and deep skillet and heat a tablespoon of avocado oil in it. Add the chopped onion and cook it on medium heat until it becomes translucent. Now ass the garlic and cook for another minute. Then add the chopped bacon and rest of the spices and stir everything together. Cook until the bacon is not pink anymore and fully cooked. Now add the kale leaves and pecans and cook until the kale is tender and spears bright green. Now turn off the stove and set the filling aside.

Now remove the roasted squash from the oven and flip with the cut side up. Drizzle with maple syrup. Now add the fillings into the squash and fill each evenly. Sprinkle with some pomegranate cheese and dairy-free cheese if you like. Serve warm and enjoy!

5. Pumpkin pie smoothie

Have you every heard of a healthy smoothie which that tastes like pumpkin pie? Nope, right? You are going to hear about it now. This smoothie is enriched with all the healthy nutrients that support fertility and is an amazing drink to fulfill your drink cravings during the luteal phase.

Course: Drink/ smoothie
Cuisine: American
Preparation time: 10 minutes

Ingredients:

- Almond milk – 1 and ½ cups
- Steamed pumpkin – 1 cup
- Steamed cauliflower – 1 cup
- Collagen protein powder – 2 tablespoons
- Organic ghee – 1 teaspoon
- Organic cinnamon (ground) – ½ teaspoon
- Nutmeg (ground) – ¼ teaspoon
- Vanilla extract – 1 teaspoon

Instructions:

Ad all the ingredients to a high-speed blender and mix until everything is thoroughly combined and appears smooth. Serve cool and enjoy!

6. Instant CBD mug cake

Instant mug cakes always seem to be a very unhealthy recipe. But you can turn it into a healthy one. It is the ultimate easy-to-make and fast cake recipe that is sweet and nutritious at the same time. It contains the goodness of cannabidiol (CBD) which is a hemp-derived substance that can help relieve PMS symptoms.

Course: Dessert
Cuisine: American
Preparation time: 10 minutes
Cooking time: 5 minutes

Ingredients:

For the mug cake:

- Paleo baking flour – ¼ cup
- Whole egg – 1
- Cinnamon coffee flavoring – 1 tablespoon cup
- Coconut oil – 1 tablespoon
- Organic ghee – 1 tablespoon
- Coconut sugar – 2 tablespoons
- Cinnamon powder – 1 teaspoon
- Vanilla extract – ½ teaspoon
- Baking powder – ½ teaspoon
- Sea salt – ½ teaspoon

For CBD frosting:

- Dairy-free cream cheese – ½ cup
- Organic maple syrup – ¼ cup
- Lemon juice – 1 tablespoon
- Vanilla extract – 1 teaspoon

Instructions:

Take all ingredients of the frosting in a bowl and mix them together by using a beater. Set it aside. Take the dry ingredients of the mug cake except coconut sugar in a bowl by sifting each of them. Transfer the ingredients into a microwaveable large mug. Take a separate bowl and add the egg, coconut sugar, cinnamon coffee flavoring, ghee and vanilla extract in it. Whisk them together until thoroughly combined.

Now make a hole in the middle of the dry ingredients in the mug and slowly add the wet ingredients into it. Use a fork to mix the ingredients together in circular motions. The mixture should be thick and wet. Place the mug in the microwave and cook for about two minutes on high. The mixture should turn into a firm cake-like appearance. Now add the cream cheese frosting on tome and sprinkle with some cinnamon and sea salt. Serve right away!

PHASE-SPECIFIC EXERCISES

The peak levels of progesterone that are reached during luteal phase can cause you to become drowsy and make your energy levels low. Therefore, it is important to not strain yourself during this time. Excessive muscular strain on your body during this time can cause cardiovascular stress and unconsciousness. This is especially common for women who are involved in strength and endurance training and live in hot and humid weathers.

If you workout on a daily basis then you can continue your workouts during this phase but try to take more water breaks in between to replenish the energy levels and give yourself time to breathe. Here are some workout options that can be beneficial during luteal phase:

Low-intensity cardio

Low-intensity cardio exercises like aerobics can help relax your muscles and relieve PMS symptoms. Such exercises include going for a walk, biking or swimming. Scientific research has proven that doing low-intensity cardio 3 times a week for 12 weeks continuously can really help regulate your hormone balance and optimize the working of your menstrual cycle especially during luteal phase.

Pilates

Pilates is a form of low-intensity exercise that involve both your mind and body. It kind of conditions you body by low-impact workouts. It strengthens your body by utilizing its core strength and helps improve your general fitness and enhances your well-being. Pilates can improve your body's flexibility and balance your posture. It relieves muscular pains associated with PMS and reduces abdominal cramps.

Intense yoga

Yoga is one of the best exercises you can do to unwind your stress and relax your body. It provides all benefits in one workout i.e., strength, rejuvenation, relaxation, and endurance. Intense yoga involves many different postures and positions that encompass your entire body. Every muscle is involved and after a 20-minute session of intense yoga, we are sure you will feel energetic and free of all those PMS symptoms and low moods associated with luteal phase.

CONCLUSION

Hormones are involved in every system, every process and every function of your body. They are the essential chemical messengers that keep your body healthy when they are in balance. A slight disproportion of this balance can wreak havoc in your body and completely tip off your physiological health on to a track of unwanted symptoms, and problematic health issues that can hinder your everyday life activities. But we are hopeful that reading this book and all the natural ways of managing hormone balance must have changed your perspective about this.

Changes in your diet, lifestyle and everyday routine is the best way to go about managing hormone imbalance in the most natural and organic way without stuffing your body with a handful of pills and capsules that come with a plethora of side effects themselves. However, nothing should be pursued without the consent of a professional health care provider. If you think you have symptoms of hormone imbalance, then consult your doctor first. Know your body's health status and nutritional requirements and only then go for a diet routine or lifestyle adjustment under the supervision of your doctor.

The journey to a healthy and balanced hormonal system is not an easy task. We know it sounds tedious and takes time but nothing is impossible if you have the will. You need to believe in yourself. Start with small steps and we are sure that one day you will make it to your goal of healthy hormones and feel accomplished.